HOLONOMIC REFLEXOLOGY

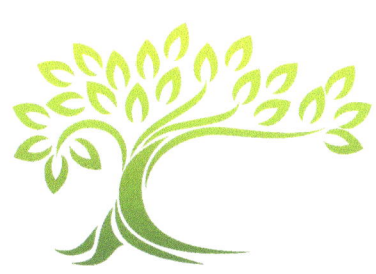

AN INTEGRATED WHOLE BODY SYSTEM

FROM

POLARITY THERAPY

Morag Campbell PTP and Phil Young PTP

Masterworks International Publishing

Published in Great Britain 2017, revised edition published in 2019 by

MASTERWORKS INTERNATIONAL

27 Old Gloucester Street

London

WC1N 3XX

England

Tel: 00353 (0)86 325 2645

Email: admin@mwipublishing.com

Web: http://www.mwipublishing.com

Copyright © 2017, 2019 Morag Campbell and Phil Young

Cover design by MWI design

Graphics: Special thanks to Michael Nolan

13 digit ISBN: 978-0-9933465-4-5

All rights reserved. No part of this book or other material may be reproduced in any form without written permission of the publishers.

Holonomic Reflexology stimulates the body's life energy currents. It is not intended to be a substitute for needed medical care. Any application of the knowledge and techniques herein are used entirely at the reader's discretion and risk.

CONTENTS

Introduction	4
Why Holonomic?	6
The Roots of Holonomic Reflexology	8
Energy	11
Holonomic Perception	24
Conscious Touch	30
Holonomic Cartography	35
Maps and Charts	51
The Astrology Connection	73
Holonomic Treatment Strategies	80
Holonomic Treatments	91
Holonomic Treatment	93
Constitutional Treatment	96
Holonomic Foot Reflexology Session	101
Diaphragm Treatment	104
Organ Treatments	106
Spinal Correspondences	118
Esoteric Correspondences	123
Final Thoughts	154
Bibliography	155
Credits	156

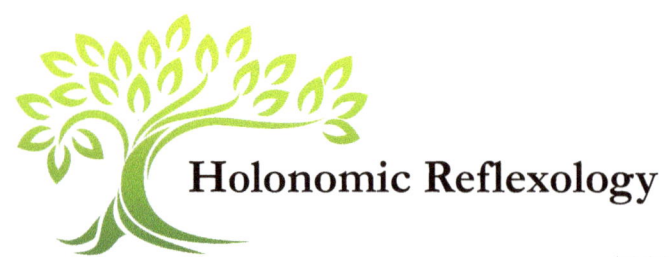

Holonomic Reflexology

Taking Reflexology to the Next Level

Introduction

The work of Dr. Randolph Stone, which we have been teaching for over thirty years, is a synthesis of many different forms of healing, which Stone integrated, through the concept that everything is energy, into a cohesive healing art which he named Polarity Therapy.

All of the approaches to healing that he integrated are still practised today as stand alone systems, but without the emphasis on the life energy. This book shares his energy based approach to Reflexology, or as it was known in his era, Zone Therapy. Building on this foundation, we have incorporated concepts derived from the physics of biological systems, as well as a deeper appreciation of the significance of ancient esoteric knowledge, into a unique approach that we call Holonomic Reflexology.

This is no ordinary Reflexology book. It focuses on the vital energy that is the matrix for life itself. When we are connected to the greater energy field that surrounds us, our energy is in abundance and flows naturally, and we can say that we are in a state of health and wellbeing. Today's lifestyle, and our divorce from a connection to the natural world and the rhythms inherent in it, takes us away from health rather than sustaining it.

Beyond the classic foot, hand and ear reflexes, there exists a myriad of reflex areas and correspondences throughout the whole body which we explore in depth. To effect true healing it is often not enough to simply work one or two reflexes. The interconnectedness of the body, where nothing exists in isolation, means that any disturbance can set up multiple areas of imbalance throughout the body. This requires a whole-body approach to fully restore health.

A human being is much more than just a body. True healing embraces all levels of body, mind and soul. Holonomic Reflexology addresses the deeper, hidden aspects of mind and soul and their related patterns of energy.

For the Reflexologist, this book will introduce a new perspective on reflexes that can be incorporated into any existing practice. The concept of working reflexes through conscious intentional touch that deeply influences the life energy will be new to many.

For Polarity Therapists, this book will re-ignite their enthusiasm for the practice of Polarity Therapy as a whole body system of reflexology that acknowledges the fundamental patterns, shapes or forms that underpin all existence.

For all bodywork therapists, the perspectives outlined in the following pages should inform, clarify and inspire a new appreciation for the rich tapestry of correspondences that exist all over the body—a true reflection of the Creator's art.

Morag Campbell & Phil Young

Holonomic Reflexology offers the possibility to touch every level of what it is to be human.

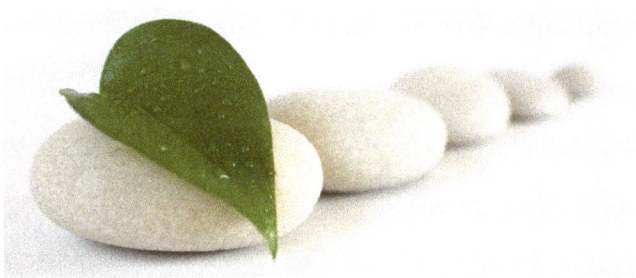

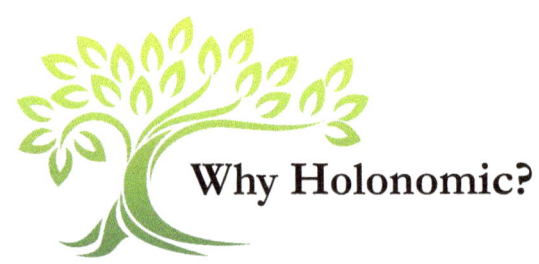

Why Holonomic?

In 1978 George Leonard wrote *The Silent Pulse*. In this book he postulated that life is rhythm, vibration and harmony. Harmonics, in a musical sense, is actually another way of understanding reflex relationships in the human body. Like many people in this period he was fascinated by the development of holograms and saw that it could offer a model to explain some of the unusual features of reality and human life. A hologram requires certain very specific technology for both its production and use. Due to certain inherent problems in the application of concepts that underpin a technological process when applied to a biological system, Leonard proposed the use of the word 'holonomic' meaning in the nature of, but not actually, a hologram.

In this same era, scientists Karl Pribram and David Bohm also turned to the science of holography to illustrate their theories, particularly in relation to mind and brain function. They theorised that the brain operates in a manner similar to a hologram, not as a single hologram but as multiple localised holograms within the workings of the brain. Their theory provided an explanation of how the brain is able to maintain function and memory even when it is damaged. It is only when there exist no parts big enough to contain the whole that memory is lost. This holographic model for human cognition is drastically different from conventionally accepted ideas.

A holographic theory of the universe connects everything with everything else and, in principle, says that any individual element could reveal detailed information about every other element in the universe. This echoes the ancient hermetic viewpoint of '*as above, so below*'. Other theoretical physicists have also postulated that our whole universe is, in fact, one big holographic projection. Holographic theory seems to run parallel with the Hindu concept of *maya* which states that everything is illusion, a mere projection that sustains the illusion of permanence.

If the human being is indeed a microcosm of the universe then this principle would certainly apply to us. We could say that human beings are indeed *holonomic*. If we take this a step further we could extrapolate that within us are all the answers to Life, the Universe and Everything.

Bohm later developed what, in essence, was seen as a new model of reality. His theory of the *Implicate Order,* as he called it, posited that wholeness is not a static oneness, but a dynamic '*wholeness-in-motion*' in which everything moves together in an interconnected process. Here is where theoretical physics is analogous with more ancient, esoteric beliefs about the nature of the universe and consciousness.

Perhaps the most important aspect of these models, as they relate to reflexes, is the argument that the hologram has the ability to store information, each small part having the ability to store all the information of the whole. The holonomic concept that every part of us may have the potential to store information about the whole of our being raises the concept of reflexes and correspondences to a new level.

The whole in the part, as William Blake said:

> *To see a World in a grain of sand*
>
> *And a Heaven in a Wild Flower*
>
> *Hold Infinity in the palm of your hand*
>
> *And eternity in an hour*

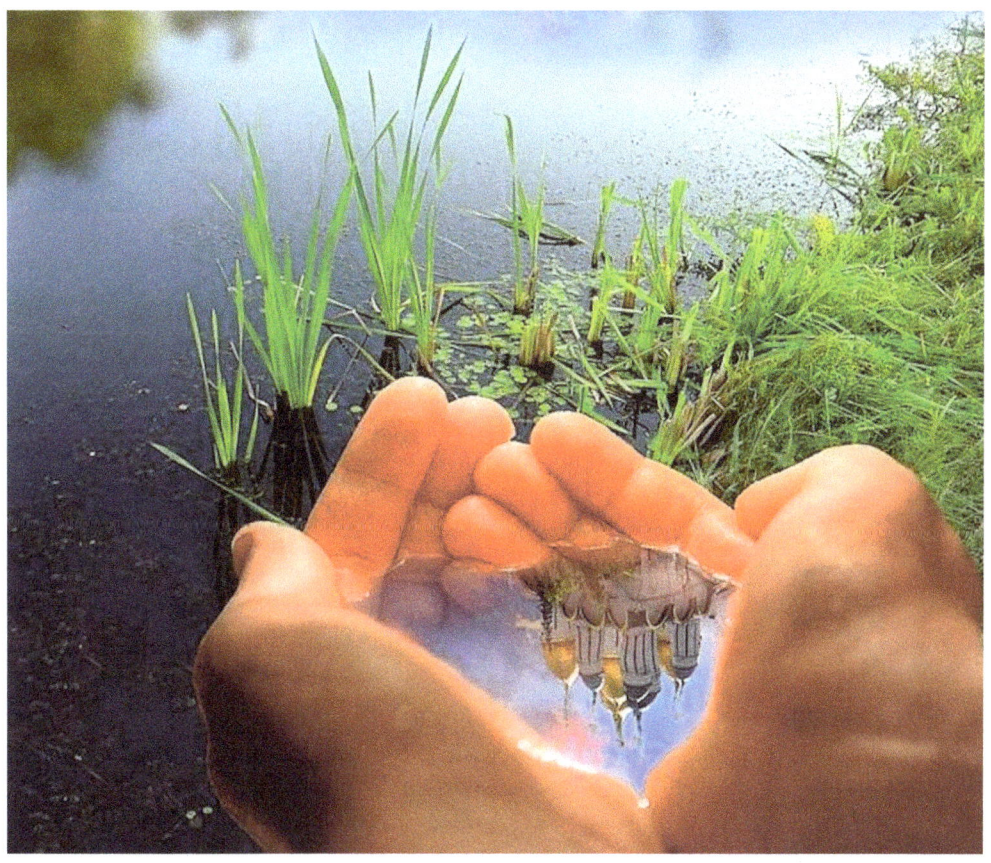

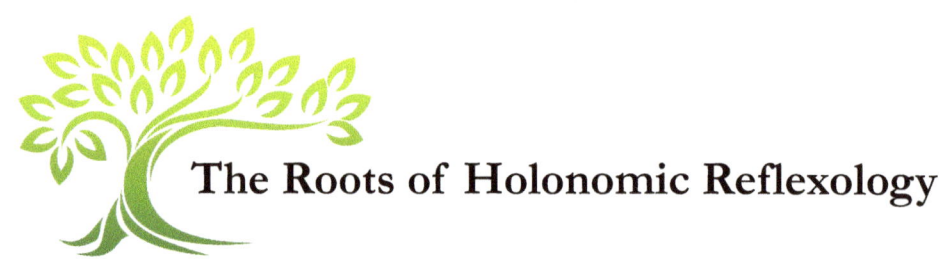

The Roots of Holonomic Reflexology

Dr Randolph Stone D.O. D.C. N.D., the founder of Polarity Therapy began exploring reflexology in 1917. He had been in practice as a doctor of manual medicine since 1914. Like many therapists of this era, he was interested in learning new techniques to enhance his work. It quickly became clear to him that reflexology worked in clinical practice. The question was how?

He explored the answer to this question for over forty years. He wrote:

> In 1917 Dr. Fitzgerald published a book, through I. W. Long and Company, called "ZONE THERAPY". This book was widely circulated and created much attention by means of the phenomenal results obtained. Zone Therapy was tried by many doctors of all schools, and it created quite a following as a new idea and approach in the healing art at that time.
> The system was unique because it did not go into hypnotism, mesmerism, suggestive therapeutics, nor into psychism. The results were obtained 'entirely' by manipulation of extremities and their reflexes in respective zones.
> But the main weak point was the lack of a scientific, acceptable foundation which could reasonably explain the modus operandi of its working and the phenomenal results obtained by some faithful adherents. For want of a better term to explain this phenomenon, it was attributed to reflexes, especially of the sympathetic nervous system, and was later called "REFLEXOLOGY".
> On closer examination, the underlying facts did not bear out a system of reflexes which could be traced by any nerve connections like the sensory and motor reflexes. In most cases the connection through nerves as reflexes, could not be established.
> *Human Reflexes* - Newsletter - September 5th 1957

ZONE THERAPY used definite areas for reflexes, but, for lack of any other explanation, supposed them to be of a more physical nature, flowing over nerve currents. However, the five lines or zones certainly do not conform to any tracing of nerves. Rather, they are a clear indication of a

much older system, known for thousands of years before physiology and anatomy were thought of.
Polarity Therapy Versus Zone Therapy - Newsletter - September 26th 1957

This older system that Dr. Stone speaks of is a naturalistic viewpoint that perceives the world as composed of life energy, a vital force present in all living things. In 1921 poet D. H. Lawrence wrote:

> I honestly think that the great pagan world of which Egypt and Greece were the last living terms, the great pagan world which preceded our own era once, had a vast and perhaps perfect science of its own, a science in terms of life. In our era this science crumbled into magic and charlatanry. But even wisdom crumbles.
> I believe that this great science previous to ours and quite different in constitution and nature from our science once was universal, established all over the then-existing globe.
> *Fantasia of the Unconscious*

From this perspective our body manifests into form first, as invisible swirling light and sound energy that then coalesces into lines of energetic force that are the matrix for the creation of the physical body.

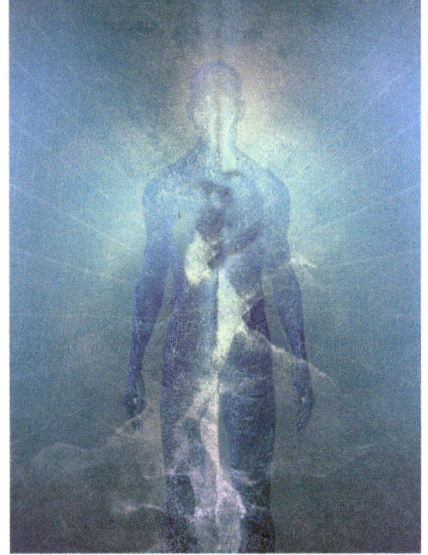

> I had used Zone Therapy and figured out a real logical foundation for it besides being just arbitrary dividing lines. My divisions are living lines of finer energies which travel in wireless waves and are latent in the body like the energies circulating in an atom.
> *Polarity Therapy* -Vol II, Book 5, p. 104

> The only answer I know is based on "Polarity Therapy" which deals with the Energy Currents and fields instead of only the end results of bones, nerves, muscles, etc.
> *Human Reflexes* - Newsletter - September 5th 1957

Dr. Stone goes on to say how these living energy currents are the essence of Vitality:

> Intelligence and control of the Mind Principle and its four derivative functions is bypassed as a sort of superstition of the past. The fact that these Energy Currents, as mentioned by the Ancients, are the very life of matter is not convincing enough for modern science to accept it. The ancient symbolism of portraying these facts to us by the simple currents of 'earth, water, air and fire' means nothing to present day science because they have never pursued this line of Energy Research which leads into VITALITY itself and is the support of all things.
> *Vital Balancing* - Newsletter - September 25th 1957

> "Reflexes are really vitality responses. Without an inner active centre or nerve ganglion, there is no response to any surface stimuli. Life or vitality (called 'Prana' in the East) is the elastic mainspring upon which all response or reaction depends."
> *Vital Balancing* - Newsletter - September 25th 1957

This vital energetic balance that Stone speaks of was his answer to how reflexology works. This understanding evolved into an exploration of the complexity of the many reflexes that emerge throughout the whole body underpinned by the movement of life energy. Indeed, one definition of Polarity Therapy is that it is a system of total or whole body reflexology.

Holonomic Reflexology embraces all of Dr. Stone's understandings of the body's reflex relationships as well as embracing other more modern understandings of the dynamics of human interaction.

> "<u>VITAL BALANCE</u>, as a practical approach to the problem of <u>life</u> and <u>health</u> is both <u>possible</u> and <u>applicable</u>. Since the Life Energy is the Builder and Architect of our body, it is also the Maintainer and Sustainer of it".
> *Polarity Therapy* - Dr. Randolph Stone - Vol II, Book 5, p. 5

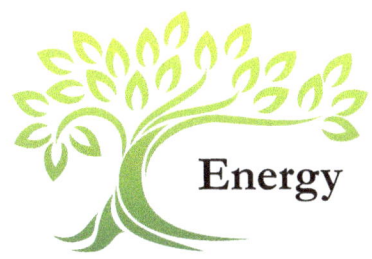

Energy

Energy or vitalism lies at the heart of Holonomic Reflexology, the practice of Polarity Therapy and many other approaches to healing. Yet, this life energy is one of the most difficult things to define simply and clearly.

Any good teacher or writer, when dealing with obscure topics, will often resort to the use of analogy and metaphor as an aid to the readers' comprehension. In our exploration of life energy, analogy, poetry and metaphor will be used but none of these are the reality of the experience of life energy.

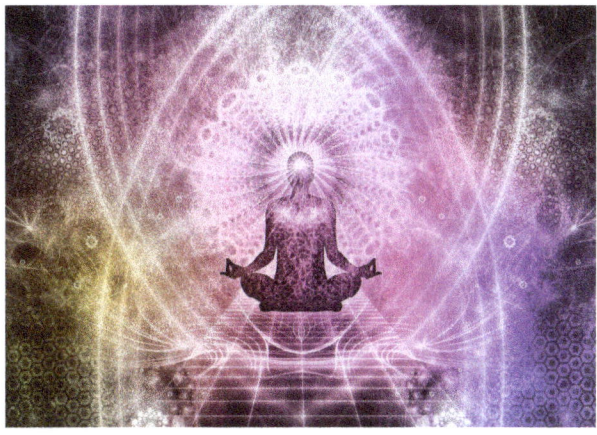

Life Energy in History

The concept of a life energy (*élan vital, chi, ki, prana,* and *pneuma*) dominated the history of medicine in the West until 1842-1845. In this period, the Herman Hemholtz School of Medicine emerged. Its primary vision was make sure that any vitalistic concepts were completely excluded from the biological sciences. The school was both reductionist and deterministic. Members of this school wanted to demonstrate that the structure and function of living beings were explainable solely in terms of the concepts of physics and chemistry. This approach to medicine was started by Du Bois-Reymond and Brücke, who in 1842 pledged their famous oath:

> "[We pledge] to put in power this truth: no other forces than the common physical chemical ones are active within the organism. In those cases which cannot at the time be explained by these forces one has either to find a

specific way or form of their action by means of physical mathematical method, or to assume new forces equal in dignity to the chemical physical forces inherent in matter, reducible to the force of attraction and repulsion".

Sadly, this reductionist trend has continued unabated in the field of allopathic medicine for the last 175 years. It is only in the field of alternative and complementary medicine, which embraces so much from ancient cultural sources such as traditional Western, Chinese and Indian medicine, that vitalism still holds sway.

The biggest issue with the reductionist approach is that it does not consider the effect of consciousness and reflective self-consciousness or self-awareness upon biological systems. Consciousness is an intrinsic component of the life energy.

Our modern understanding of life energy in the West derives largely from the work of C.W. Leadbeater, Annie Besant, and A.E. Powell. From these authors and their books such as; *The Etheric Double, Astral Body, Mental Body and Causal Body* and *Occult Chemistry*, we have the terms, 'etheric energy' and 'etheric double'. The etheric double is the body of life energy which some like to call the subtle body.

Dr. Stone, the founder of Polarity Therapy, from whose work Holonomic Reflexology is mostly drawn, was very familiar with this terminology and understanding. However, he was also deeply influenced by the emerging atomic science and modern Western physics and its electromagnetic energies.

What is in a name?

Our word 'energy' dates back at least to Aristotle in his use of the word 'energia' meaning, activity, action, operation' and from Heraclitus who used the word 'energon' meaning active, working. In ancient Greece, the sense of both terms could be encapsulated as actuality, as opposed to another Greek word 'dynamis', which is potentiality. It is interesting to note that in modern English we often use these two words together when, for example, we refer to someone as having 'a dynamic energy' meaning they have high vitality, thus blurring any real distinction.

In modern Western physics energy is simply defined as the ability to do work. Energy in physics obeys certain laws. These laws are usually called the three laws of thermodynamics. Simply expressed these three laws are:

1. The conservation of energy.

2. Entropy always increases.

3. The entropy of a system approaches a constant value as the temperature approaches absolute zero.

Entropy, which is a core concept, is simply the measure of disorder and randomness in a system. British scientist C.P. Snow created a humorous way to understand the three laws as: (1) you cannot win (you can't get something for nothing because matter and energy are conserved.) (2) You cannot break even (you cannot return to the same energy state because entropy always increases) (3) you cannot get out of the game (because absolute zero is not attainable).

The publication of the book *Energy Medicine – The Scientific Basis* by Dr Jim Oschman, 2000, revised 2016, was a landmark. In it, the author reviews all the latest research and findings on all the different levels of electromagnetic energy in the body according to modern physics. Yet, fundamentally, it is not a book about the vital life force or etheric energy.

> "Our science is a science of the dead world. Even biology never considers life, but only mechanistic functioning and apparatus of life".
> *Fantasia of the Unconscious* - D.H. Lawrence - 1921

Life energy obeys a different set of laws than the three laws of thermodynamics listed above. Indeed, from the perspective of the life energy, entropy is decreasing, meaning that the function of life energy brings more order not less to a system.

What is Life Energy?

From a naturalistic pre-scientific perspective, life energy is that which our five senses, that is to say, what we can see, touch, taste, feel and hear—tell us is the difference between a living and a dead body. If you consider a human being when they alive; they are conscious and communicative, they take in food and drink and excrete the waste material, they move about, they breath in and out, their heart beats and there is a warmth to their body. When they die the first thing you notice is the cessation of breathing, and the general lack of all other movement, then you realise that consciousness is no longer present. Finally, if you come closer, you may realise that the heart has stopped and the body is beginning to cool.

This simple experience forms the basis of almost all descriptions of life energy. In essence, nearly all of these definitions come down to saying that life energy is movement and aliveness. The word 'aliveness' in this context relates to consciousness itself and the way in which our thoughts, emotions and feelings are fundamentally linked to life energy.

The poem below expresses this most eloquently:

> —And I have felt
> A presence that disturbs me with the joy
> Of elevated thoughts; a sense sublime
> Of something far more deeply interfused,
> Whose dwelling is the light of setting suns,
> And the round ocean and the living air,
> And the blue sky, and in the mind of man:
> A motion and a spirit, that impels
> All thinking things, all objects of all thought,
> And rolls through all things.
> *Lines Composed a Few Miles above Tintern Abbey* - William Wordsworth - July 13th, 1798

Being conscious means being alive yet, where is consciousness itself located? Modern science would have us believe it is an epiphenomenon of the physical brain yet, from a naturalistic perspective, consciousness is a meta-physical phenomenon that exists both within, and outside of, the physical body. Perceptually, it is as if consciousness is both in and not in the physical body. Yet it is consciousness that lies behind the physical bodily impulses to move and breathe.

Where is the Life Energy?

In exploring the life energy you will often come across such statements as 'energy flowing in the body' and simple variations of this phrase. This is a fundamental error of thinking. Life energy does not flow in the physical body in the same way, for example, as the blood flows in that body. It is not like a hand going into a glove. Subtle energy, which is non-physical in nature, cannot flow in a physical body.

This idea, which is rooted in the dominance of our physical sciences, has led to endless confusions when people have looked for the physical medium through which the life force can flow. It has given rise to such ideas as the chakras (the step down transformers of life energy) are related to either the endocrine glands or nerve plexus and that the life energy itself flows in the blood or cerebro-spinal fluid. Similarily, the flow patterns of life energy are often related to the nervous or vascular systems.

All of these theorisations and explorations are simply an attempt to reconcile and resolve the antithesis of vitalism and mechanism—because if a physical medium for the life energy is found it has been reduced to a mechanistic concept and there is no more conflict. Such a reductionist approach takes the life energy out of the realm of the spiritual, mysterious and unseen and firmly places it into the realm of the mundane. All this speaks to the power of the reductionist, mechanistic viewpoint and its dominance in Western culture.

The reality is that energy can flow in the physical body provided that by this phrase we mean the electromagnetic or kinetic energy that is active within the physical body, being both of the same nature and existing in the same realm or plane of existence.

Subtle life energy can flow, or be active, but only in a body or form that is within the realm in which life energy and consciousness exists. So, we can say that life energy can flow in a body that is elsewhere than the physical body. That body is often called a subtle body, etheric body or body of life energy.

In ancient times, the naturalistic viewpoint on this issue began to speak of other worlds, planes or realms of existence. The simple experience that gives rise to this concept is that of sitting by a river bank, on a sunny day, perhaps thinking of catching a fish to eat, and placing the fishing rod partly in the water as you bait the hook, you notice that your rod, which intellectually you know to be quite straight, appears to bend in the water. If you try to touch the rod where you see it, it is not there! Somehow you cannot believe your senses. A good spear fisherman in the ancient world knew that if he threw the spear where he saw the fish, he would not have fish for supper. Even the simple action of putting your arm into the river creates an interesting duality of experience, you can feel your arm to be straight and yet your eyes inform you that it is distorted. There is where you see your arm and where you feel it and they are not the same, yet they are definitely related in your consciousness.

Of course, our modern understanding of the behaviour of light moving through different mediums explains this phenomenon. Yet from the naturalistic perspective this sense of something being slightly out of place when an object is in a different medium creates the basis for understanding that the life energy and its body are related to the physical body but a little out of place or out of phase.

Ultimately, scientific research into life energy is doomed to fail as the only thing a scientific experiment, being based in the physical realm, can measure is the *effect* of life energy on the physical body not the actual energy itself. The effects of energetic disturbance can be registered in the physical realm using sophisticated physical measuring devices but we can only infer from this what might be happening at a subtle level. It cannot be measured directly.

Life Energy – Formative

There is an understanding that the life energy is a formative force. It organizes life on the physical plane. By way of an analogy, you can view this organising process as functioning much like the way that a magnet organises the alignment of iron filings placed within its magnetic field. This formative aspect of the life energy means it can be thought of as a 'dynamis'—a knowledge holder—a directing, intelligent force. This aspect of the life energy as both an intentional or volitional force and an intelligent one implies, ultimately, that it is a conscious energy. Some might say it is an expression of the mind or consciousness of God stepping down in to different planes of reality.

Life Energy – Adaptive

In his seminal book *The Stress of Life* Dr. Hans Selye posited the existence of an adaptive energy in the human body writing, "The term adaptation energy has been coined for that which is consumed during continuously adaptive work, to indicate that it is something different from the calorific energy we receive from food; but this is only a name, and even now – almost thirty years after this hypothesis was first formulated – we still have no precise concept of what this energy might be". As a Western trained doctor Selye was only looking in the physical body for the source of this adaptation energy when its real source is the life force. The life energy in the human body is as we posited earlier a continuously formative energy but it is also the basis of the body's ability to adapt to the stresses and strains of living. We use our life energy to cope with all the demands and challenges of everyday life physically as well as mentally and emotionally. The more life energy we have and the better it flows the more animated we are. We deal with stress and strain, whatever its source and nature, more effectively when we are deeply animated by an abundance of free-flowing life energy.

> "All pain is a break in this vital Energy Current. All pleasure is a free, full flow of it".
>
> *Polarity Therapy* - Dr. Randolph Stone - Vol I. p. 68

The Experience of Life Energy - Movement

Life energy is often perceived directly as streaming pleasurable sensations in the body, an experience that clearly gives rise to fluid based models of energy currents. A typical experience of energetic activation, following a session based upon energy work, might be like the one below as described by American actor Orson Bean:

> I walked out the door and down the hall. It seemed as if my feet barely touched the carpeted halls. I came out into the air and crossed the street into the park. I looked up into the sky over the East River. It was a deeper blue than any I had seen in my life, and there seemed to be little flickering pin-points of light in it. I looked at the trees. They were a richer green than I had ever seen. It seemed like all my senses were heightened. I was perceiving everything with greater clarity. I walked home feeling exhilarated and bursting with energy. That night I went to work at the theater and got through my show somehow. I didn't know if I was good or bad. I got home sometime after midnight, and knew there was no remote possibility of going to sleep. Far from settling down, the energy coursing through my body had increased as the night went on, moving rhythmically up and down

from head to toe. There was no doubt in my mind that it was orgone energy or whatever the hell name anyone wished to give it. It was like nothing I had ever felt before and I knew that I had tapped into the strongest force in the world.
Me and the Orgone - Orson Bean - St. Martin's Press, New York 1971.

Most people have experienced some level of streaming energy when it is triggered by a sense of awe or through music that touches them deeply. An interesting aspect of these powerful life experiences is that the hold of ego consciousness is loosened by them. The ego often perceives these streaming sensations as an uncontrollable power within, just as Orson Bean alludes to in the last sentence above. Hence, a certain level of release in the grip of the ego is an essential aspect of the ability to experience these streaming sensations.

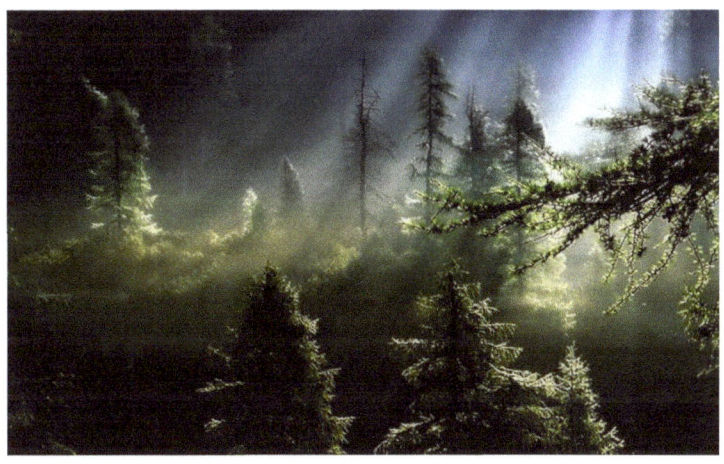

THERE was a time when meadow, grove, and stream,
   The earth, and every common sight,
      To me did seem
   Apparell'd in celestial light,
The glory and the freshness of a dream.
It is not now as it hath been of yore;—
     Turn wheresoe'er I may,
      By night or day,
The things which I have seen I now can see no more.

These quotes from Wordsworth's poem *'Intimations of Immortality from Recollections of Early Childhood'* speak to the life of the child, when the ego is less well formed and the experience of the life energy is not filtered or suppressed.

The experience of the life force so powerful in youth often fades as a child becomes an adult.

> Our birth is but a sleep and a forgetting:
> The Soul that rises with us, our life's Star,
>   Hath had elsewhere its setting,
>   And cometh from afar:
>   Not in entire forgetfulness,
>   And not in utter nakedness,
> But trailing clouds of glory do we come
>   From God, who is our home:
> Heaven lies about us in our infancy!
> Shades of the prison-house begin to close
>   Upon the growing Boy,
> But he beholds the light, and whence it flows
>   He sees it in his joy;
> The Youth, who daily farther from the east
>   Must travel, still is Nature's priest,
>   And by the vision splendid
>   Is on his way attended;
> At length the Man perceives it die away,
> And fade into the light of common day.

The Experience of Life Energy - Consciousness

There is a well-known method for experiencing the life energy between the hands, as a field of energy, which involves simply rubbing the front and the back of the palms vigorously together for about 30 seconds. Then opening and closing the hands (stretching the fingers and palms) rapidly for about a minute, followed by holding the hands about 6 inches or 15 centimetres apart, with the fingers stretched gently, and slowly moving them back and forth toward each other with a small movement of no more than 1/2 inch or 1 centimetre. Usually, a distinct sensation is experienced between the hands.

It is important to do the movement slowly and make sure that the shoulders are relaxed. It may take up to 2 or 3 minutes of slowly moving the palms before anything is felt. In some cases, the exercise may need to be repeated a couple of times a day for no more than 3-5 minutes at a time, over two or three days, before something is experienced.

The typical sensations people report is that it feels like a pressure between the hands, like pushing on a balloon. Some people say that it feels like repulsion or the feeling you get when pushing the two north or south poles of a magnet together. Some say that it is a sticky sensation. Whatever you feel, the general experience is that there seems to be something between your palms. That something is a field or area of intensified life energy.

What have you actually done in this process? In essence, you have simply done several unusual repetitive movements that have intensified your conscious awareness of your hands and the space in between. You could, in fact, say that you have created a field of consciousness between your palms. So could life energy be conscious awareness? Most of the time consciousness is a diffuse process that we pay little attention to. Right now, as you are reading this, how much awareness of all the various parts of your body do you have? Probably relatively little. Yet, as soon as you ask yourself this question your awareness of your body increases. You become more conscious of it and your life energy is more active. The linkage is so profound that you are almost inescapably drawn to the conclusion that life energy is consciousness.

From the ancient naturalistic perspective, the whole world and everything in it is conscious—plants, rocks, trees, animals, man and the Earth itself. The only difference is the degree or amount of consciousness in each and, in the human being and some so-called higher animals, the possibility of the development of self-consciousness—the consciousness of being conscious. Equally, you could say that the whole world and everything in it is energy.

When you are more conscious and aware of a particular part of your body, you have more information about what is happening in that area, so the life energy functions as an information carrier. As the life energy moves throughout the body, it functions as an internal communication network.

If the presence or absence of a consciousness life energy is something that defines the difference between life and death, it must be concluded that it is also a *continuously* formative life giving energy.

Life Energy in Health and Disease - Coherence

We could perhaps as easily have drawn upon such theories as quantum entanglement and non-locality as a way of explaining the underlying dynamics of reflexology. However, from an energetic perspective the holonomic model offers, in some ways, a more concise explanation. One aspect of the holonomic model is that when you look at the creation of a hologram using light, that light source must emit a coherent beam. This is why a laser is used in the creation of a hologram. Lasers emit coherent light.

Light emitted by a flashlight or an ordinary household light bulb, is incoherent. This means that the photons emitted are of many different frequencies and are oscillating in different directions. It is not a stream of light but a radiant expanding field.

Coherent light is a beam of photons (particles of light) that are all at the same frequency and move in the same direction. A beam of coherent light such as that emitted by a laser will not spread and diffuse. In lasers, the light waves are identical and in phase, which produces a beam of coherent light.

When we think of the energy channels or pathways in the body you can imagine that, in some cases, the energy waves run through them in a disordered way with a certain amount radiating out away from the channel. By working with the energy in the channels directly through conscious energetic touch, we mimic the effect of the tube within which coherent light develops in a laser. Within the cavity of the laser tube the beam of light is reflected back and forth along the central tube, until the waves of light become coherent. In terms of the energy, as we engage with the energy in the channels, moving it back and forth, it too, begins to become a coherent energy flow. When a therapist places their hands on the body they act like the reflecting areas in a laser but in this case it is the energy that is being reflected back and forth rather than light.

Just as the coherent light in a laser is an amplification of the initial light source and can be used for cutting and burning so to the creation of coherent energy in the channels in the human body can cut through blockages and illuminate deep recesses where the normal radiant energy has not been able to reach.

Creating a coherence within the body's energetic system is the key to healing.

Energy Disturbance

The absence of the life energy is an extreme state that marks the end of life. However, throughout life there are constant challenges to the free movement and play of the life energy. If the movement of the energy is disturbed, or if there is not enough of it, or if it is compromised in some other way, then its ability to interact with and support the function of the physical body both formatively and adaptively is damaged and dis-ease will arise. The fundamental premise of all energy based healing modalities is that if these disturbances of the life energy are resolved then health will return.

There are at least three commonly used metaphoric models for describing the manifestation of life energy within a human being. These metaphors are light, sound or water based. In terms of light, people with abundant life energy are spoken of as being glowing and radiant and if the energy is compromised they can be dark, overshadowed, dull or burned out. In relation to sound, the energy is resonant, the person is tuned in or of sound mind and when disturbed there is discord and disharmony. In terms of water, someone could be overflowing with good feelings or simply be 'in the flow', when disturbed their mind could be foggy or they could be bogged down or mired in difficulty.

In terms of the specific characteristics of the movement of energy, the most commonly used metaphor is based upon fluid dynamics, there is talk of energy flowing or being blocked and that can, over time, become stagnant, or that there is only a trickle of energy in the system. There may be too much in one place and too little in another. All these descriptions can be seen in nature as the behaviour of water. Whilst it is a valid model, it does not lead to very sophisticated interactions with the client's energy system. Alongside the use of the fluid model, in which, when the energy gets blocked, it requires unblocking and when there is an imbalance, you essentially siphon the energy from where it is in abundance to where there is a depletion, you should also think of the movement of energy as being affected by diffusion, damping, deviation or deflection, loss of impetus, a break or no pathway. The strategies for the resolution of these disturbances are outlined below.

Diffusion ⟶ Refocus

(Diffusion is a spreading out and depletion of energy, think of a river delta.)

Damping ⟶ Remove resistance

(Damping is a suppression of energy perhaps caused by another higher frequency of energy.)

Deviation ⟶ Redirect

(A blockage may cause a deflection of energy.)

Loss of impetus ⟶ Strengthen source

(Think of a car, when for some reason the engine stops—the car slowly comes to a halt. Its impetus to move is gone. There are numerous possibilities implied in strengthening the source of that movement. Has it run out of petrol? Has the electrical system failed or the engine management computer system froze? In terms of the life energy, strengthening the source would normally imply work on the chakras and the higher frequencies of mind energy i.e. working with emotions, beliefs, values and attitudes.)

Break of continuity ⟶ re-connect

(A break is conceptually similar but not identical to an 'energy block'. A block may allow the movement of a percentage of energy around it, a trickle effect, whereas a break allows no movement.)

No Pathway ⟶ Create or find a new pathway

(In some cases, where there is a break it may not be possible to reconnect the ends. In that case, a new pathway will need to be found.)

If you find that you cannot get energetic coherence or perhaps do not even feel any energy response at all, then you can begin to think of what might be causing the lack of response. Is there a leaking away of the energy somewhere or is the energy diffused, being damped down, deflected, or is the flow broken somewhere?

The best general strategy to remedy the situation is to lessen the distance between your contacts until you feel the energy between your hands as a coherent flow. Then, begin to increase the distance, until you feel the reaction in the areas of correspondence that you wish to activate. This process will help to overcome any damping or diffusion of the energy flow. In the case of deflection or deviation, again use less distance between your contacts and then move your hand laterally left or right until you feel the direction in which the energy is being deflected, then use your intention to re-direct the flow.

If you sense that there is a leakage or loss of impetus somewhere then strengthen the source by working the elemental centre that relates to zone or astrological triad of the organ you are sensing as having a problem (see p. 79). In some cases, it is enough to simply work the foot and hand reflexes for a lot longer than normal until you feel the energy responding.

A true break in the energy flow is not that common. However, if in the process of reducing the distance and leading the energy to where you wish it to go, you find that you cannot get it beyond a certain point, you have a couple of options. Firstly, you could focus on the area which you cannot get the energy to flow through by making contacts over the area left/right, top/bottom and front/back using both hands. Work on feeling the energy becoming active in the area then re-check to see if you can now get the energy to flow through this area. Secondly, you could actively, via your intention, divert the energy around the area and then on to where you wish it to go, effectively creating a new pathway.

Healing Energies - Etheric and Electromagnetic Energy

Dr. Stone wrote that there are both electromagnetic energies and etheric life energies in the human being. It is undoubtedly true that when a practitioner of any kind of manual therapy puts their hands on a client's body there are specific and, ultimately, fully mappable, electromagnetic interactions between the two physical bodies. Yet these interactions, as healing as they are, take place at a physical electromagnetic level. They are related to the mundane level of physical existence. Indeed, any manipulation of the soft tissue in the body will produce profound changes in the electro-magnetic field of the body. This can affect everything from muscle tension patterns and structural balance to cellular activity.

Dr. Stone's energy maps are his illustration of movement and pathways of etheric energy. However, if you look at Dr. Stone's depiction of the energy flows they do look uncannily like the electromagnetic field lines around a magnet. It begs the question as to what the relationship is between the etheric life energy and the electromagnetic energy.

There is a two-part answer. Firstly, the law of attraction and repulsion operates in both the subtle etheric plane and at the electromagnetic level. There is an understanding that the subtle life energy in its formative aspect in some way governs or controls the activity of the physical plane with its electromagnetic energies. Many people, including Dr. Stone, believe that the etheric energy is the blueprint for the behaviour of energy at the physical level. So, there should be a certain similarity in the drawings of etheric energy and the electro-magnetic energy field around a magnet.

Secondly, it is important to remember to whom Dr. Stones writings were addressed. In his books he often writes: 'The Doctor…' his readers being doctors of manual therapy, such as osteopathy and chiropractic, just as he was. He used the then-current scientific terminology taken from modern physics to make his ideas on energy more acceptable to his peer group. One only has to remember that diagnostic and treatment approaches using electromagnetic radiation were only coming into general usage in the mid 1940s exactly the time when Dr. Stone began writing his books on Polarity Therapy. In spite of his usage of the term electro-magnetic in his charts, he mostly appears to use this term as a metaphor for the patterning and behaviour of life energy. He seemed quite clear on the differentiation in the quote below:

> We are too much interested in taking apart things which are produced by these Energy Currents, and we forget their mode of flow and manifestation. Ancient symbolism is rejected, but our modern symbolism of chemistry, of atomic science, of electrical potential measurement, etc. are regarded highly and form the essential part of our technical education. It never dawns on us that there could be a science or an education beyond these material aspects, which leads directly into Vitality and Mind Energy Balance. We are eager to form new systems from new discoveries, but we shy away from the Unit itself, which expressed itself in this way. That road, which leads into higher fields and aspects of the mind, where Life itself becomes intelligent, is steered clear of and considered as hearsay of the past.
> *Vital Balancing* - Newsletter - September 25th 1957

In Holonomic Reflexology, and in Polarity Therapy, the focus is on the life energy and the subtle rather than electromagnetic dimension of existence.

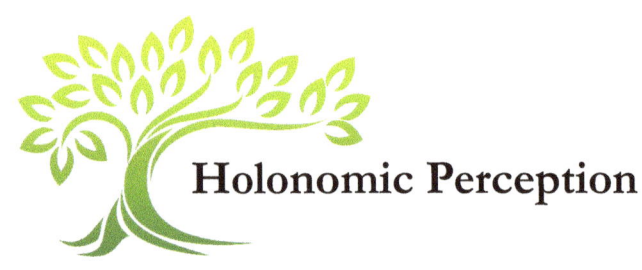

Holonomic Perception

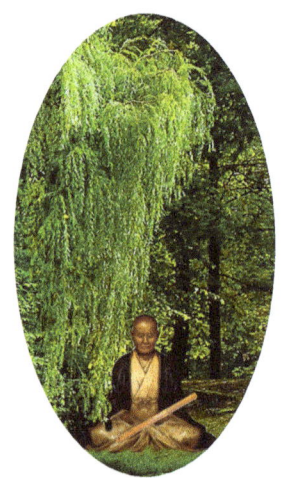

In a quiet glade, beneath the swaying branches of a gnarled willow sits a solitary figure. In his hand is a length of bamboo. Closing his eyes, the man slowly lifts the bamboo to his lips and we become aware that it may be something other than a simple piece of wood. Taking a deep breath, the man expels the breath from his lungs into the bamboo and the air is filled with sound. Suddenly, the true potential of the bamboo is revealed as his breath moves through it.

Holonomic perception involves the ability to notice the smallest of detail whilst also being aware of the whole, the 'everything' that is occurring, noticing the changes, the variables and the potential in every experience.

It is possible to utilise the techniques outlined in this book without conscious energetic awareness, in a mechanical and formulaic way, but to do so, without holonomic perception, is to miss the detail, to merely see the bamboo and miss the melody.

The actual perception of the life energy is both a simple and complex matter. In one sense it is clear that if life energy is consciousness, then the perception of life energy is related to the process of being conscious of consciousness or being aware of being aware. To perceive life energy requires an expansion of your consciousness.

Right now, as you are sitting reading this book how much are you aware of your body? Are you aware of the tension in the musculature of your hand as it holds this book? Are you conscious of the movements of your eyes as you read the words on the pages? Are you aware of the pressure of your buttocks on the seat of the chair? Are you conscious of your feet on the ground or of your legs curled beneath you if you are sitting more casually? Having answered these questions, is the content of your consciousness wider than before you answered these simple questions? Are you feeling more vital, more alive, more present?

Holonomic perception of the life energy in the body is different from the simple perception of the energy in and between your hands that we explored in the chapter on energy. It is a more complete experience that takes in your whole body and that of your client. In effect, you and your client blend in one homogenous field of awareness where information is being exchanged constantly.

It is important to begin with the experience of the energy between your hands and to be totally comfortable and familiar with that focused expansion of your awareness. The deepening of simple physical awareness is a unique gateway to the subtle energetic realms of existence. As an experiment, place one of your hands comfortably on your thigh and let the palm and fingers mould to the contour of your body. Allow yourself to be aware of the texture of your clothing, and then experience the weight of your hand on your thigh. Is there a perception of warmth available to you? Is there a movement of air over or around your hand? Is it easier for you to perceive these things if you close your eyes? What is the difference between the sensations in the thigh that you are touching compared to the other? Do you sense something happening inside the thigh that you are touching? If you sense a difference in your thigh, is that perception coming to you via your hand or is it an awareness from inside your thigh more directly or both? Is there a difference in awareness between both your legs in a more general sense?

All these questions are posed as examples of how to deepen your experience. Fundamentally, after a while, you begin to shift from purely physical experiences to other unusual sensations that are, in essence, the experience of life energy moving in and through your body. When you are comfortable with this experience try it with a partner, placing your hand on their thigh and going through the same deep observational process.

Ultimately, the exploration of the perception of energy can take years. There are so many different possibilities in terms of the way energy is experienced. Typically, for most people, the sensations are usually pulsation, vibration or a magnetic push and pull. However, anything is possible. It is a unique individual experience and depends entirely upon one's consciousness.

As a final stage, when you are familiar with this process within your self and then with a partner, experiment with expanding your awareness outward to include the room that you are in, being aware of the eight corners of the room and the space enclosed within it. As you expand your awareness fully in this way, you may notice your attention flitting from one place or aspect to another, within the complete experience. If this is the case, see if there is a way you can expand awareness such that you are aware of everything, all at once, without any movement of your conscious awareness.

This kind of instantaneous all at once holistic or holonomic perception is a profound level of information processing. Essentially, information is coming to our consciousness via our five physical senses. What we can hear, see, touch, smell and taste. The first three of our senses, the auditory, visual and kinaesthetic, and their subtle counterparts in the realm or plane of life energy, are the most important when it comes to the perception of energy. Apart from their basic function, there is a modulation of the activity of each of these three senses, which is less well known. Each of these senses can have either a broad or narrow focus as well as being focused either internally or externally. As an example, one of the authors of this book experiences the life energy most clearly by having very little visual input (closed eyes), a very broad external auditory focus (like listening to an orchestra) and a variable kinaesthetic perception that shifts back and forth from a narrow internal focus to a broad internal and then to a broad external focus. You can see that reflected in the type of questions posed in the life energy perception exercise with the hand on the thigh.

Whilst much has been made of the role of the three primary senses (auditory, visual and kinaesthetic) in many different therapeutic approaches, the influence of internal/external and broad/narrow focus upon them has received much less attention. Yet they are perhaps more important. The distinction between internal-external allows for the perception of both time and space. As a young child develops their perception of internal and external they become able to understand both time and distance (i.e. how long is it until Christmas and how far to Grandfather's house). The concept of "weak psychological boundaries" is just another way of saying a person has difficulties with differentiating between internal and external focus.

The balanced use of broad-narrow focus is not common in the Western world. Indeed, in the West there is an emphasis on narrow focus, on specialisation. The child at school is told to concentrate, meaning to focus down onto the task at hand. Those who use broad focus are often thought to be dreamers and underachievers, they don't 'pay attention', they never 'focus on anything', but this distinction, which is widely used in the Orient and by tribal and first world cultures, has a great deal to do with the experience of wisdom; the ability to 'step back and see the big picture', 'hear the music of the spheres', or 'feel the greater connection of all things'.

An exploration of the examples below will help you to expand your Holonomic perception and to understand what type and balance of sensory experience expands your consciousness of life energy most effectively.

Auditory

>**Internal Broad**: Imagine or remember the sound of a roomful of noisy people, listening to a flock of birds singing or the roar of a stadium crowd during a game.
>**Internal Narrow**: Imagine or remember the first violin in a piece of music, the squeak from a door or a small animal scurrying.
>**External Broad**: What is the total sound of your present environment? All the sounds. Is there a motor running? A fan? Insect noise?

External Narrow: Pick just one of those sounds in your immediate environment and listen intently to it, what is its character? Then pick a different sound.

Visual

Internal Broad: Imagine or remember an impressive vista, a sunset or sunrise for example, or the longest train you have ever seen or an army of 5,000 men marching.
Internal Narrow: Imagine or remember looking at the very tip of your pen as you write or the point where a highway or motorway vanishes into the distance.
External Broad: See as much as you can of the room you are now in, both to the sides as well as up and down, without moving your gaze. How far in each direction?
External Narrow: Pick the smallest thing (.5 cms or .25 ins or less) you can now see (within your immediate area) and examine it carefully. What colour is it? Is it rough, shiny, smooth, pointed?

Kinaesthetic

Internal Broad: How is your general physical well being—head to toe? Do you feel warm, cold, full, tired? Be aware of your heartbeat—can you sense the pulse in your fingers and feet?
Internal Narrow: What is the sensation in your left big toe, your right knee and left ear? Which is warmer, your right or left hand?
External Broad: How tightly are your clothes fitting at the moment? Remember the feel of jumping into cold water; the heat of the summer sun on your body?
External Narrow: Is there a movement of air over the back of your right hand? How is the fit of your right shoe?

Do the hand exercise explained in the chapter on energy again and explore how the use of any of the above alterations of your perception can enhance the experience of the energy between and in your hands.

Therapeutically speaking, the use of broad focus is very important in the practice of Holonomic Reflexology. It is, of course, possible for the therapist to simply focus down on the energy and its response where the hands are in contact with the client's body and, once a release and shift is felt there, to consider that the work is done. However, it is always important to understand how these local changes are affecting the whole of the client's energy system. This requires the use of broad focus.

This broad focus will inevitably go beyond the client's body and lead to the inclusion of the perception of the therapist's own energy as part of a larger whole. This conjoint energy system, composed of that of both the client and the therapist, is governed by the laws of complexity.

The Therapist & Client—A Complex Adaptive System

In Holonomic Reflexology, the client and the therapist are perceived to form a unique, or combined energetic entity, a conjoint system that behaves as a complex adaptive system. Complex adaptive systems have some unique characteristics or properties, the key ones being that they are:

- **Emergent**: Rather than being planned or controlled, the individual parts in the system interact in apparently random ways. From all these interactions patterns emerge which inform the behaviour of the agents within the system and the behaviour of the system itself.
- **Co-evolving**: All systems exist within their own environment but they are also part of that environment. Therefore, as their environment changes they need to change. As they change, they change their environment. Then, as the environment has changed they need to change again, and so on.
- **Sub-optimal**: A complex adaptive system does not have to be perfect in order for it to thrive. It only has to be slightly better than its competitors and any energy used on being better is wasted energy.
- **Self-organising**: There is no hierarchy of command and control in a complex adaptive system. There is no planning or managing, but there is a constant re-organising to find the best fit with the environment.
- **Nested**: Most systems are nested within other systems and many systems are systems of smaller systems.
- **At the Edge of Chaos**: A system in stable equilibrium does not have the internal dynamics to enable it to respond to its environment and will slowly (or quickly) die. Systems exist on a spectrum ranging from equilibrium to chaos. A system in chaos ceases to function as a system. The most productive state for any system to be in is at the 'edge of chaos' where there is maximum variety and creativity, leading to new possibilities and a much better chance of long-term survival.

Complex adaptive systems have within them:

- **Requisite Variety**: The greater the variety within the system the stronger it is.

- **Connectivity**: The ways in which the individual parts in a system connect and relate to one another is critical to the survival of the system. The relationships between the individual parts of the system are generally more important than the parts themselves.
- **Simple Rules**: Complex adaptive systems are not complicated. The emerging patterns may have a rich variety, but like a kaleidoscope the rules governing the function of the system are quite simple.
- **Iteration**: Simply put, iteration means repetition. In terms of complex adaptive systems each repetition builds upon the result of an earlier one. A rolling snowball, for example, gains on each roll much more snow than it did on the previous roll and very soon a fist-sized snowball becomes a giant one. Even very minute changes in the initial conditions can have significant effects after they have passed through the emergence-feedback loop a few times. This so called 'butterfly effect' is the sensitive dependence on initial conditions in which a small change in one state of a system can result in large differences in a later state.

The most significant characteristics in the context of Holonomic Reflexology are that the journey the therapist and client take toward health is an evolutionary one, with the therapist and client mutually connected and freely exchanging information. The avoidance of repeating patterns of behaviour and interaction is of deep importance, both therapist and client need to consciously embrace variety. In this ongoing journey, sometimes the smallest change can snowball into a major shift. The movement towards health is a complex and sometimes confusing process existing on the edge of chaos. Health is not a state of being but a process of living with unstable equilibrium and a less than perfect result is often good enough.

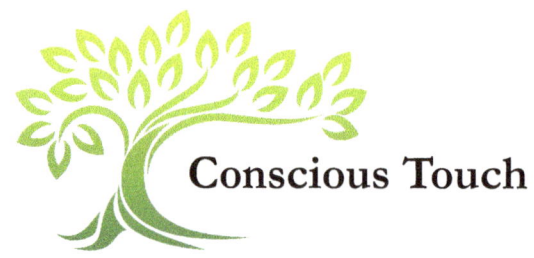

Conscious Touch

Just as in classical reflexology, the primary medium of interaction with the client in Holonomic Reflexology is through the hands and physical touch. The touch used is not, however, merely the application of pressure to the tissues but a conscious touch which engages with the tissues of the physical body *and* the life energy and requires the therapist to be totally present and focused in their hands. Conscious touch is not the mere application of technique; it is not just doing something to the body, rather it is the recognition that we are energy beings making contact with another being of energy, able to converse in a language that is so much richer than mere words, powerful as the spoken word can be. It is a deeper, more intimate connection, an unspoken dialogue consisting of the flow of consciousness itself. Consciousness that is connected to the greater field of consciousness of all life on this planet, with its multitude of nuances and resonances.

Conscious energy based touch is a process of communication, of information exchange. Sensing the life force specifically through the hands or finger tips entails a clearing of any internal dialogue in the mind and, in part, a narrowing of consciousness, focusing down on the subtle movements and sensations that are occurring on and beneath the surface of the skin.

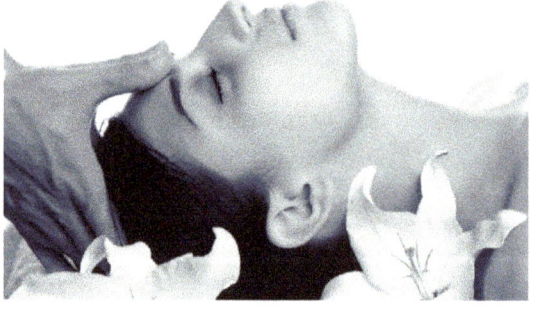

When we focus on the physical sensation beneath our fingers and hands we can observe, for instance, that the area may be tense, the tissue may be cold, spastic and unyielding or swollen and spongy. There may be a degree of pain or discomfort even under the most sensitive pressure application on our part. These observations are important to the therapist but they are just as important to the client as it brings their awareness to the area and the sensations they are experiencing. Through conscious touch an unspoken dialogue ensues between the therapist and the client which some people have also described as a kind of dance. As the touch elicits subtle changes in the client, the therapist's touch changes to acknowledge that change and then waits for and responds to any further communication that may take place. The body and energy response always informs our next action. As in any communication, listening and waiting for a response is absolutely essential. True communication is in the feedback.

The nature of the actual perception of the life force in the subtle body via the hands or fingers is completely subjective. It may, as we mentioned before, be recognised as temperature differences, tingling, vibration, pulsation, magnetic pressure or indeed any sensation that is beyond the easily recognised feedback normally experienced from just physically touching the body.

The body will usually recognise and respond to conscious touch by reducing tension and easing discomfort as well making other adjustments to bring both body and mind back into a state of ease and comfort.

If there is little or no response then gentle stimulation with the pad of the thumb or fingers with a circular motion that spirals deep into the tissues is advised. This mode of touch is designed to energetically 'wake up' the area by stimulating the life force with the clear intention of releasing the energy that may be held there or invite more energy into the area so that it may once again flow unimpeded. Our clear intention is crucial. We are sending a message via our conscious awareness, through our hands, that 'invites' the body to respond.

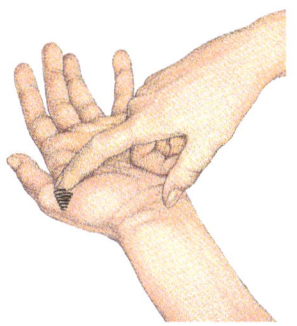

After a moment or two of this stimulating touch pause and gently hold. It is important to keep the hands soft and relaxed but contactful. In most cases, the body/mind will respond to this deeper stimulating touch, the tissue will soften, fresh blood and energy will flow into the area and any pain will disperse. A lack of reaction means that the body is unable to respond because there is a holding elsewhere. It then becomes crucial to establish where in the body the energy is compromised and to free it. At this stage, a broad focus on the whole of the client's energy system allows us to assess where the disharmony and lack of connection is so that we can adjust our focus.

Responses to Conscious Touch

It is important to say something about the kind of responses that the use of conscious touch in the practice of Holonomic Reflexology can elicit.

Entranced

Most commonly, this touch will encourage the client to go into a state of deep relaxation. During periods of deep relaxation several trance state phenomena can be observed. The eyes may sink deep into the skull as the tension leaves the small muscles around and behind the eyes, or the eyes may move rapidly under the eyelids with movements that are reminiscent of REM sleep patterns. There may also be some lacrimation.

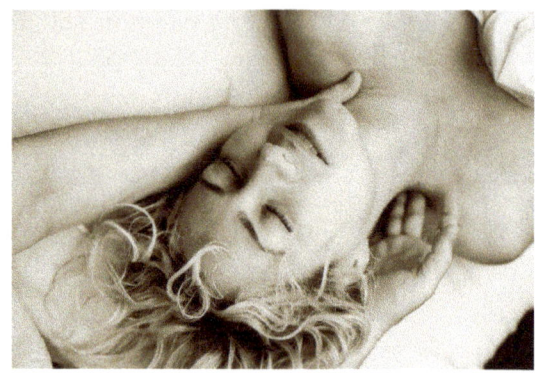

The pallor of the face often changes and the cheeks redden slightly. This may also be accompanied by repetitive swallowing. All these signs indicate the client has shifted into an altered state of consciousness. They will often dip in and out of these states during a session and it is during these deep trance states that the healing potential of the body is activated. The conscious control has been temporarily held at bay and the deep, unconscious well of resources can come into play without interference.

The Body Responds

A softening of the tissues under your hands is a strong indicator of the effectiveness of your touch. Any softening of the tissues is always accompanied by an increase in blood flow and a re-vitalisation of the area. When we make a conscious contact with the body we are connecting with a living, intelligent, sophisticated biological system, which responds to the impulses that it receives from our hands by re-organising and evolving in response to that stimulus. Your hands and the client's body are involved in a constant dialogue, where information is continuously passing back and forth, leading to adaptation and change along the way. With sensitivity and conscious intent, we are able to highlight the tension, stagnation, emotion etc. that is trapped in the tissues and energy, then given that information, the body will, whenever possible, move toward a higher level of organisation and function.

In order to achieve that re-organisation, the body will often exhibit various easily recognisable responses. A common reaction is a shift in breathing as there is often a need to draw more oxygen into the body to cleanse and re-vitalise. This is accomplished by deep sighing or yawning, sometimes quite uncontrollably for several minutes. Changes occurring in the nervous system are accompanied by a shift to deeper breathing and this can act as a physical guide as to when to release your contacts and move on.

Over breathing, which can occur as the client seeks to stay with a powerful sensation or emotion can lead to a condition called tetany. This condition comes about as a result of the blood oxygen/carbon dioxide levels becoming unbalanced. Should this occur, the client can experience numbness and tingling, especially around the mouth and arms and, if it carries on for any length of time, the muscles of the face, neck, arms and hands can become rigid. This can be extremely alarming for client and therapist alike. The simple solution is to encourage the breathing to return to a more natural level. You can do this by placing your hand on the client's chest and encouraging them to breathe more slowly until a more normal, calm breathing pattern is re-established.

Occasionally, the body will begin to shake or jerk. Jerking of the limbs is often seen when an impulse to action, such as the desire to reach out and touch or move away from a situation, has been suppressed and over time has become a locked pattern within the nervous system. As the body relaxes that pattern is released. The shaking can be limited to a specific area of the body or spread until the whole body is shaking and the teeth may even chatter. This reaction is frequently accompanied by a drop in body temperature and signifies a strong release. It is usually enough to simply cover them with a blanket and wait for the process to subside.

In general, there is no need for the client to inhibit these kind of movements. However, should the client become anxious then stop the bodywork and encourage them to get up, move around and shake themselves to discharge the neurological impulse.

Frequently, during a session there is an increase in peristalsis, as the parasympathetic nervous system, commonly referred to as the 'rest and digest' aspect of the autonomic nervous system, becomes activated. This is completely normal despite most client's embarrassment at all the gurgling sounds. Occasionally, the client may have a sudden need to urinate or evacuate their bowels immediately after a session.

Localised sweating can occur in the areas being worked or sometimes the client will break out in a sweat from head to toe.

Some clients may feel extremely heavy and drained at the end of the session. This is because the body has been taken to a level of relaxation that is well below that which is normal for them. This new level of relaxation is often misinterpreted as a loss of vitality and energy until the client becomes acclimatised to it.

The Energy Responds

The client may also experience intense heat throughout their entire body as the energy begins to flow more freely and powerfully. A cold reaction, like cool water trickling within the body, is often a result of the release of old congested energy, which has been held near the surface of the body through excess tension, flooding back to its source. These reactions tend to be of short duration and cease when the energy flow normalises.

A common energetic experience is the sense of a subtle vibration throughout the whole body. This is often accompanied by streaming or flows of sensation from the top of the body downward. There may also be a feeling of pulsation, either of the whole body or in just one part. These sensations can be deeply pleasurable.

Emotional Release

These physical and energetic reactions can often be accompanied by various emotional expressions such as tears and laughter. The client may also feel euphoric, as if they are 'floating on air' and experience a new level of well-being.

Sometimes a client can feel overwhelmed by strong emotions, in which case suggesting that they inhibit the expression could be appropriate. For example, if a client is crying excessively, a soft, relaxed hand placed on their chest, accompanied by a simple comment such as, "It's okay, you can stop now. Remember, you can always come back to these feelings at another time". This will both calm and reassure.

All these reactions are the client's way of releasing and re-balancing and pay tribute to the effectiveness of the session. Everyone being unique, individual clients will react in different ways and not everyone will experience all these responses.

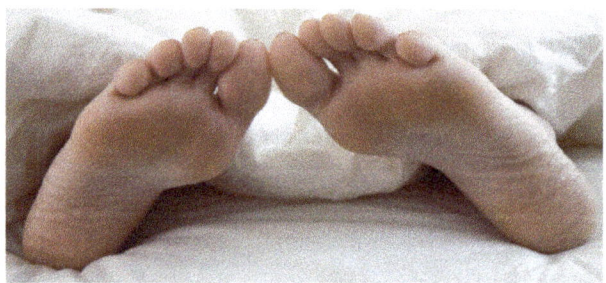

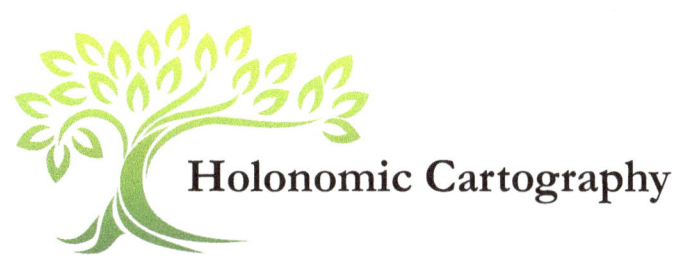

Holonomic Cartography

If the life energy in the human being is the answer to how the stimulation of reflexes and correspondences in the body can create such powerful change, then the more fundamental question is, why do so many reflexes and correspondences exist? The answer to this question lies in Plato's phrase:

God Geometrises Continually

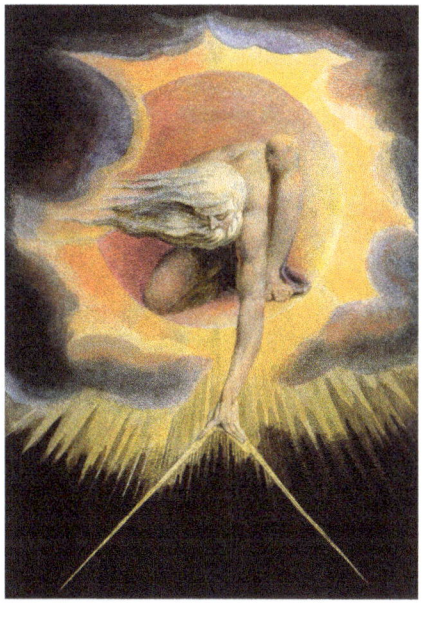

Humanity's greatest gift is the ability to create; everything from magnificent architectural buildings to an eclectic array of electronic devises, has come from human imagination. There is, it seems, a continuous outpouring of creative juices into the world. Humans seem to be encoded with a creative imperative, an evolving process towards creative change.

At the beginning of any creative endeavour, after the initial creative spark, comes a process of design, of planning and the formulation of blueprints; blueprints that define the structure and the function of each individual creation. Is it then such a tremendous leap to accept that the natural world too is an expression of the Creator's mind and imagination; that the natural world too has blueprints that define its structure and function? Blueprints written not in ink or digital code, but in mind energy. A thought or idea in the mind of the Creator. The word idea, which derives from ancient Greek, in modern usage means simply a 'thought'. However, it was used by Plato to mean 'an eternally existing pattern of which individual things in any class are imperfect copies'. This idea or creative mind energy is also known as 'pattern energy' and from it comes all the forms of the natural world.

In speaking about pattern energy, Dr. Randolph Stone wrote:

> Mind Energy and its geometric patterns of design were the blueprints of creation. It has been truly said, "God geometrizes". Everything created has proportion, balance, purpose and use. If man can make such blueprints which are mental creations, should not God, the author of all design be

the superior in this art? And is His creation less real than man's designs and patterns?
Human Reflexes – Newsletter - September 5, 1957

Another name for a blueprint is a map. The word cartography comes from the Greek χάρτης khartēs, 'papyrus, sheet of paper'; and γράφειν graphein, 'write' and is the process of making maps. To create a cartography of the human being we need to understand the fundamentals of map making, the underlying cartographic process. Cartography combines both science and aesthetics and has, as its fundamental premise, that reality can be modelled in forms that communicate information. In essence, a map is a form of language, a graphic language. It presents information in a way that is easy to understand. At their core, maps are visual expressions of measurements.

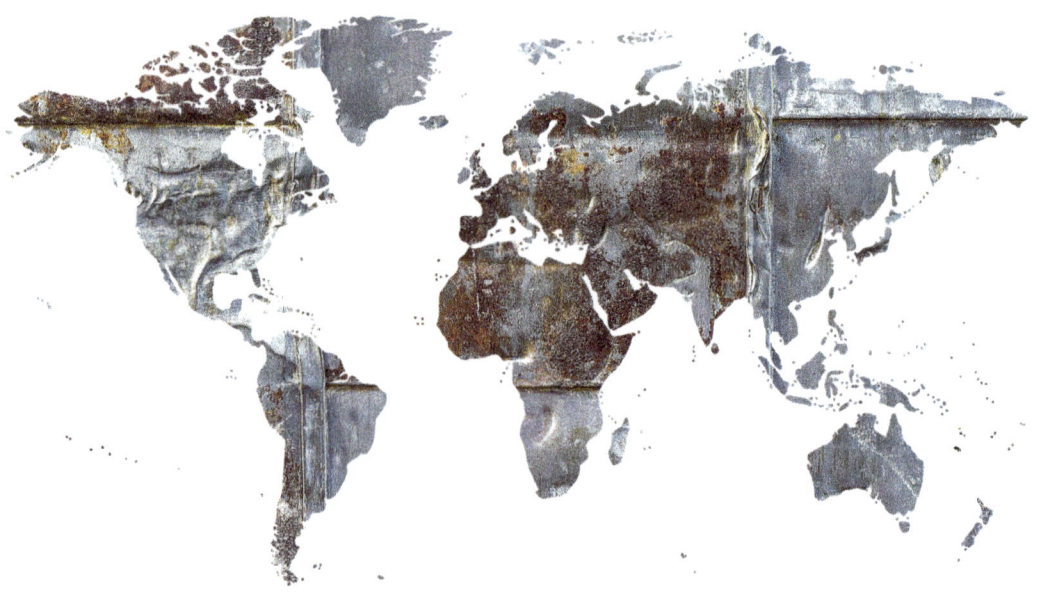

To design and build any type of structure or to map a new land, humans have evolved what we now call geometry. geo- 'earth', -metron 'measurement'. Geometry is that part of mathematics which is concerned with shape, size and position of figures and the properties of two and three dimensional space. It essentially deals with length, breadth, height and volume and can be said to be the study of points, lines, planes, surfaces, angles, curves and solid figures. Classically, this is referred to as Euclidian geometry, the study of which was of the greatest importance to the people of ancient Greece and Egypt. It is important to note that in Plato's statement he says, "God Geometrises Continually" which alludes to the concept that we have already mentioned, in the discussion about energy, which is that all the various frequencies of energy exert an ongoing formative effect throughout life.

> "There are primal pattern energies and fields in our makeup, which are as true and essential to our function and life as a blueprint is to a well laid out structure or a mechanical design. These pattern energies are a fine, wireless variety of the nature of mind substance and emotions in their various step-down functions as currents and waves. These patterns are the designs and the unseen builders in our body and in Nature everywhere. The original pattern in God's design is in the seed power of each thing according to its kind".
>
> *Health Building* - Dr Randolph Stone - p. 104

Points Of View

The fundamental key to the cartographic or map making process that lies behind the creation of the maps in Holonomic Reflexology is perspective.

The reflex maps are derived from all the different perspectives that can be taken when looking at the human body. When we view any object we are seeing it from only one perspective. Walk around that object and we get a new perspective from each differing angle of view.

Anatomy books show illustrations (or maps) of the different systems of the human body. There are maps of the skeletal structure, the muscles, the organs, the nervous system etc., each being a different perspective upon the physical body.

Books on healing may show maps of all the various meridians of Chinese acupuncture or the subtle energies of the human chakra system and the layers of the aura. Again all these maps are simply different perspectives on the human energy system.

The many reflex maps in Holonomic Reflexology come about because of the differing perspectives you can take when exploring the relationship of the whole and the parts. When Dr. Stone looked at the body from all the different perspectives available to him, he found and mapped a rich tapestry of correspondences. These perspectives are informed by certain geometric principles.

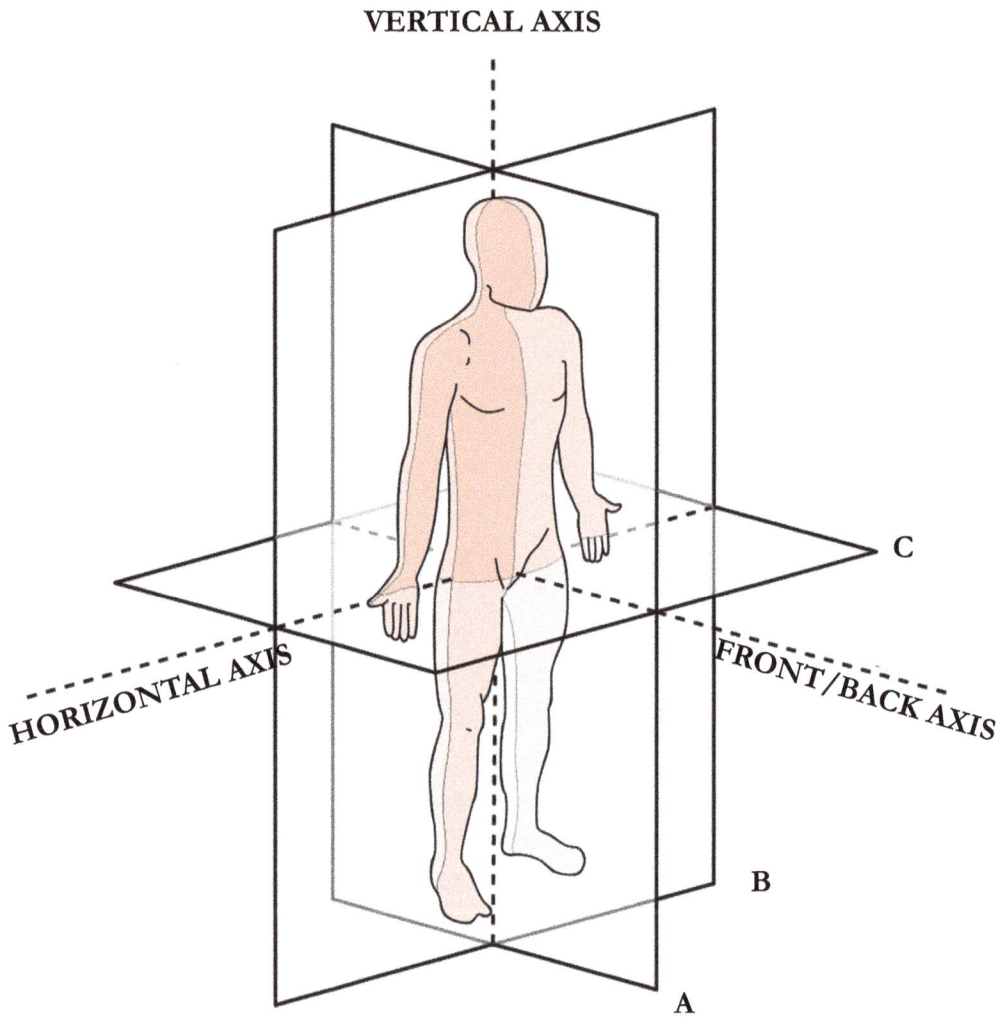

Geometry of the Human Body

The principles of geometry apply to the human body as it is an object that exists in three dimensional space. It has tri-axial geometry, that is to say, it has a top and a bottom, a front and a back, and a left and a right side to the body. The illustration above shows the three axes and the three planes of the body where A represents the Sagittal plane; B, the Coronal plane and C, the Transverse plane.

Correspondences

The energetic blueprint that both creates and sustains the physical form of the human body obeys all the same geometric principles that are seen in the forms of the natural world and the universe as a whole.

There are three geometric relationships which are important in terms of the correspondences in the body. These are Reflection, Translation and Proportionality. Specific correspondences are classified as being either reflected (or mirrored) or translated. Proportionality is always present.

Proportionality

All correspondences in the body have a proportional relationship. This is simply a way of talking about the coordinates of any point or area in three dimensional space and the way it relates or corresponds to other areas. This aspect of geometry is usually referred to as analytical or Cartesian geometry.

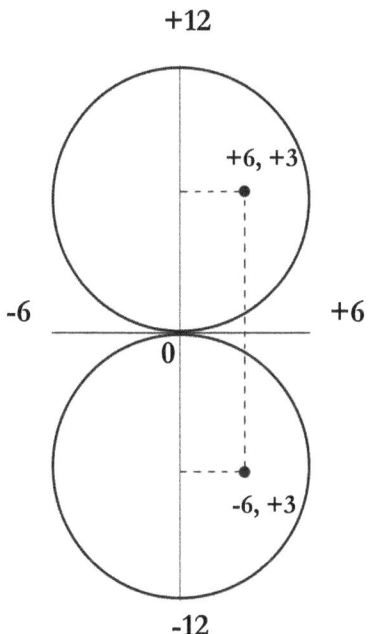

For simplicity, consider a two dimensional example with two circular objects of equal size placed in relation to a vertical axis of −12 to +12 units and a horizontal axis of −6 to +6 units.

A point in the upper circle that relates to +6 on the vertical axis and that relates to +3 on the horizontal axis will, when reflected downward through the horizontal axis be in the lower circle but its co-ordinates will be different.

The reflected point will still be at +3 relative to the horizontal axis but will now be at −6 relative to the vertical axis. An exact reflected co-ordinate relationship.

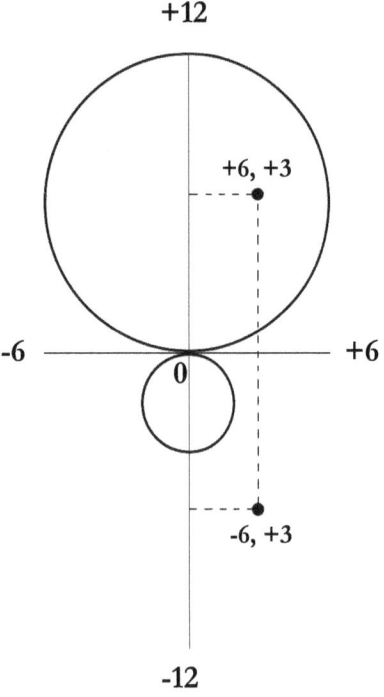

The problem is that, in relation to correspondences in the body, many of the related areas are not of the same size. This means an exact co-ordinate mapping, as we described on the previous page, is impossible. Where you have unequal sized circles, as the diagram opposite shows, the lower being much smaller than the upper, the same point at (+6,+3) in the upper circle when reflected down through the horizontal axis will not be in the lower circle.

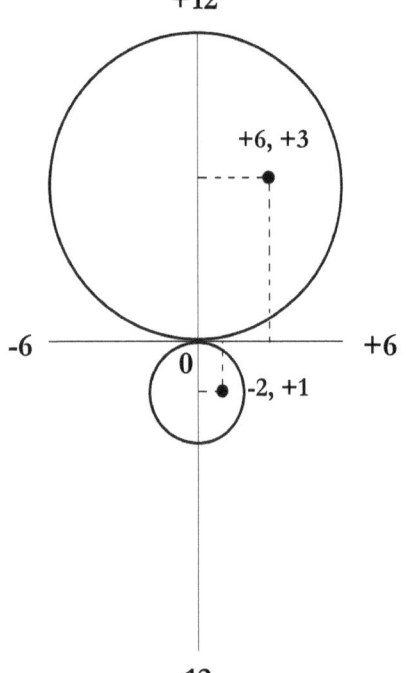

However, it is possible to reflect that point in the upper circle proportionally down into the lower circle. If the lower circle is exactly 1/3 of the size of the upper circle, the points at +6,+3 in the upper circle will be, by proportion at −2,+1 in the lower as shown opposite. The point is located by proportion.

This type of geometry is very precise.

When applying the concept of proportionality in a session, practitioners will most likely think either in terms of fractions i.e. it is half way down the body and a quarter of the way across the right side or in percentages as 50 % down and 25 % across.

Reflection

The geometric relationship called reflection or mirror symmetry is perhaps the most fundamental aspect of perspective.

A structure displays symmetry, or is symmetrical, if it can be divided in half, creating two pieces that are mirror images of each other. Two dimensionally, a line of symmetry is an imaginary line that divides a symmetrical object into two mirror image halves. In three dimensions, a plane of symmetry is an imaginary plane that divides a symmetrical object into two mirror image halves.

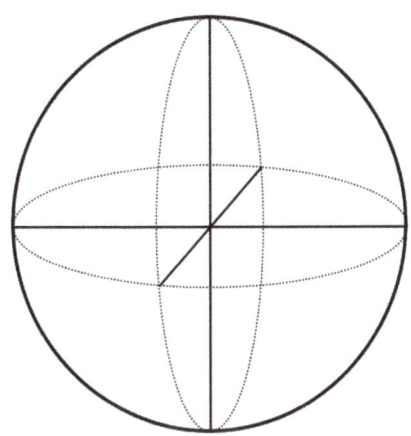

Reflection or mirror symmetry is a term used to describe any function that reflects an object an exact distance but in reverse order through a plane, axis or point of reflection

Numerically reflection would be expressed as

1 2 3 4 | 4 3 2 1

OR

1
2
3
4
―
4
3
2
1

In a three dimensional object such as a sphere there can be mirror symmetry through any of the three planes. Correspondences by reflection appear spontaneously through the sagittal, coronal and transverse planes. A sphere can have infinite lines of symmetry.

The geometric mirror symmetry that is so clearly demonstrated when looking at the front and back of the body are the basis of many reflected correspondences in the human body. In relation to reflection through the coronal plane and through the many possible transverse planes, when there is no clear geometric mirroring, proportionality is always used to map the reflected correspondences. They are reflected *proportional* correspondences.

> "Symmetry is a vast subject, important in both art and nature. Mathematics lies at its root, and it would be hard to find a better one on which to demonstrate the mathematical intellect".
> *Symmetry* - Hermann Weyl - p.145

Mirror Symmetry In Man And Nature

The geometric relationship called reflection or mirror symmetry is perhaps the most fundamental aspect of perspective. When looking at the human body we can clearly see that it has a matching left and right.

A structure displays symmetry (is symmetrical) if it can be divided in half, creating two pieces that are mirror images of each other. A line of symmetry is an imaginary line that divides a symmetrical object into two mirror image halves. The symmetrical aspect of the human body is what gives rise to mirror correspondences.

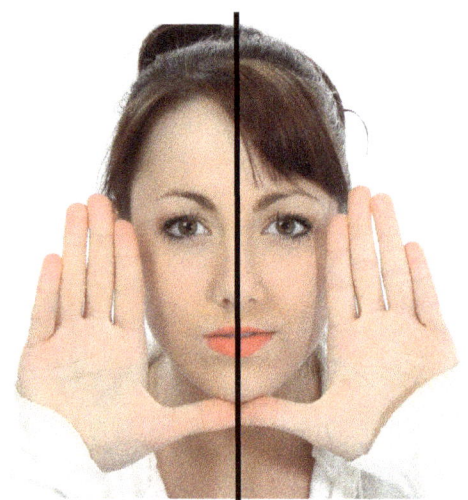

Front View

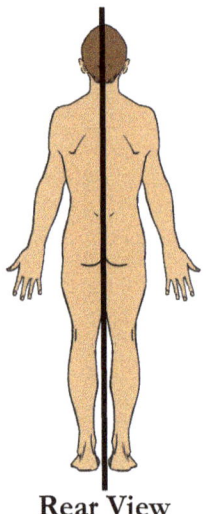

Rear View

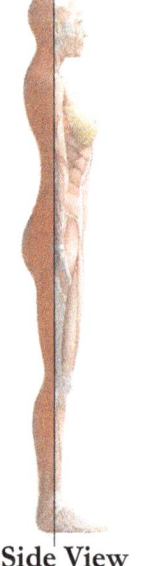

Side View

The properties of mirror symmetry and focusing on the whole or the part are also true when taking a rear view of the body.

When viewing the body from the side there is no obvious mirror symmetry between the front and the back of the body.

> "Man is all symmetry, full of proportions, one limb to another, and all to all the world besides. Each part may call the farthest brother, for head with foot hath private amity, and both with moons and tides".
>
> George Herbert
> (1593-1633, English priest and poet)

> "First, what is symmetry? How can a physical law be "symmetrical"? The problem of defining symmetry is an interesting one and we have already noted that Weyl gave a good definition, the substance of which is that a thing is symmetrical if there is something we can do to it so that after we have done it, it looks the same as it did before".
> Richard Feynman 1963

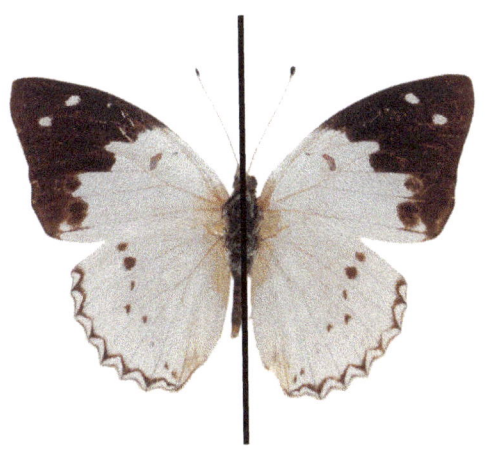 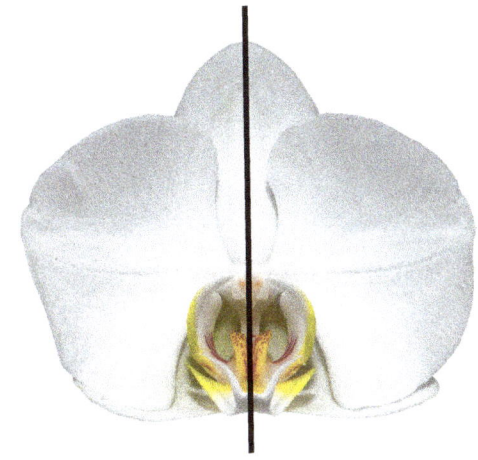

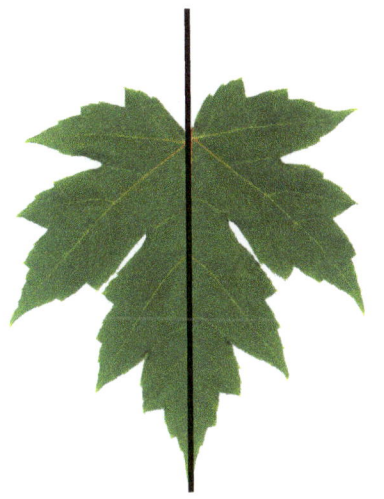

Mirror symmetry is present throughout the natural world. Although perfect symmetry, that is to say exact symmetry is rare, it is clear that overall symmetry exists to add balance and function to the organism.

Translation (Projection)

Translation is a term used in geometry to describe a function that moves a point or object a certain distance in a specific direction. A good example of this is the way that we 'cut and paste' on a computer to produce an exact replica. When we speak of translation in respect to correspondences, we mean that any point or area on the body is moved in a specific direction and for a certain distance. It is not rotated or reflected, it is simply slid in a certain direction. Translation utilises not a line of symmetry, as there is no mirroring, but a line of transformation over which the object is projected.

Line Of Transformation

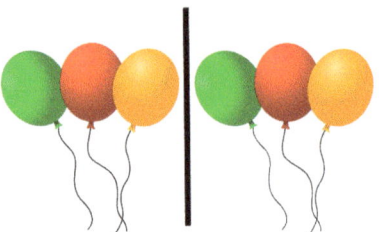

The direction in which a translated area moves is dictated by the direction of the various flows of energy in the body thus translated areas can slide up or down, left to right, front to back or diagonally.

Translation (Projection) In Man And Nature

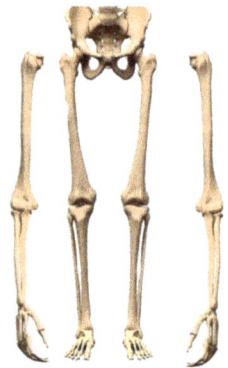

Translated correspondences may be the same size or we may need to use proportionality to map the exact corresponding area in the body.

Translation in the body occurs most obviously in the limbs. The single humerus bone of the upper arm is directly translated to the single femur bone in the thigh, the radius and ulna bones of the forearm are translated to the tibia and fibula of the lower leg and, of course, the hands with the five digits are translated to the feet and five toes. They occur in the same order as distinct from the previous examples of mirror symmetry where the order is reversed.

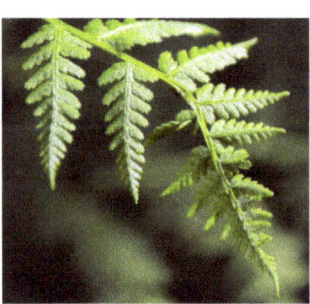
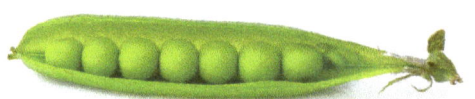
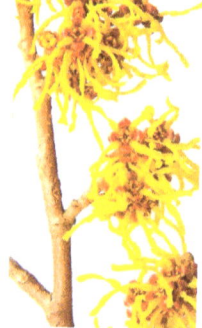

In Nature translation can be seen in the peas in a pod, the repetition of the witch hazel flowers and the branches of trees and plants.

Perspective

Holonomic reflex maps use a multitude of different perspectives to create the maps of correspondences. One such perspective is the fact that everything has a middle and two ends. If we take a stick for example, it clearly has a middle and two ends. If we take that stick and cut it in half, each half also has a middle and two ends, and no matter how many times we divide the stick, each part of the stick still has a middle and two ends.

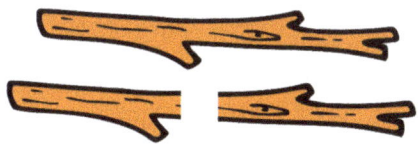

In addition to noticing the mirror symmetry then, it is possible, for example, to focus on the whole body or just a part of it.

Looking at the human body then, we can clearly see that it has a top (the head), a bottom (the feet) and it naturally hinges at the hip joints, so in this case, a line through the base of the pelvis and hips is the middle. This is one geometric perspective on the whole.

However, if we take a different perspective and dispense with the limbs and just focus on the torso, then the top is the head, the bottom now becomes the base of the pelvis and the middle is now located at the diaphragm.

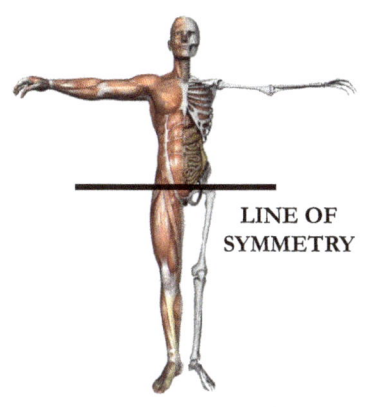

LINE OF SYMMETRY

This illustrates the establishment of varying top/bottom relationships depending on the perspective taken.

Even though there is no mirror symmetry between the top and bottom of the body regardless of the perspective taken there is a reflected proportional relationship. In the upper figure opposite, there is a correspondence between the head and the feet. In the lower figure, the head has a reflected proportional correspondence to the lower pelvis.

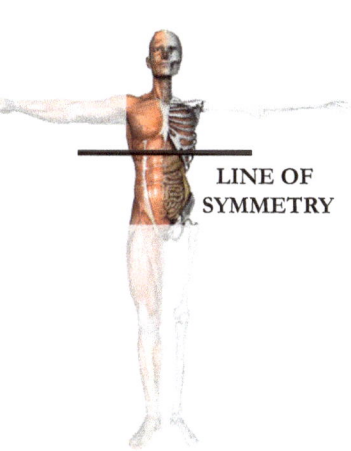

LINE OF SYMMETRY

Symmetry Of Form

Yet another perspective open to us is that of Symmetry of Form. We immediately notice a structure's shape and size when we look at it. The shape of an object helps us to identify it. The shape also helps us distinguish it from other objects. Objects which have a similar form or structure have a resonance to each other. We could say that they have the same fundamental structural blueprint or energetic signature.

Structures in the body have an energetic resonance or correspondence to other structures of similar contour, shape or form. In the human body, for instance, it is easy to see repeating patterns in the formation and structure of the skeleton. Thus the structure of the arm is the same as the structure of leg. This means that there is a direct correspondence between them.

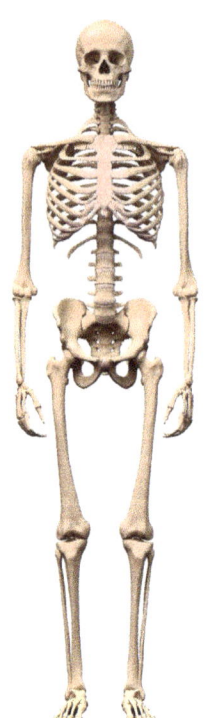

Examples of Skeletal Correspondences

The Hyoid bone and the Patella

The Humerus and the Femur

The Radius and Ulna and the Tibia and Fibula

The Elbow and the Knee

The Wrist and the Ankle

The Sacrum and the Sternum

The Hand and the Foot

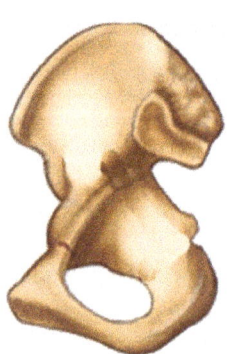 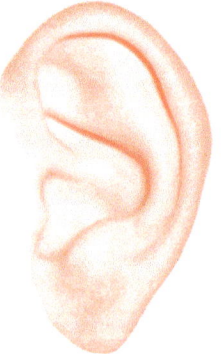

Yet another important relationship is that of the ear and the similarly formed innominate bone of the pelvis. Tension in the TMJ will have its reflection in hip tension and vice versa.

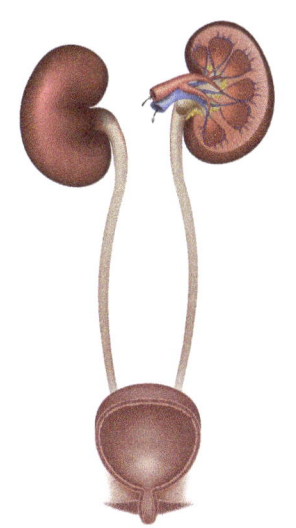 A repeating pattern of 2 similarly shaped organs that end in a single structure is a common theme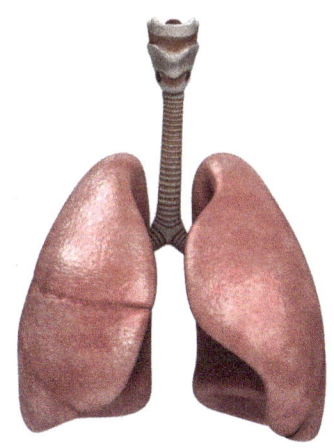

Examples of Organ Correspondences

Hemispheres of Brain and the Spinal Chord

The Lungs and the Trachea

The Kidneys and the Bladder

The Ovaries and the Uterus

The Testes and the Penis

Creative use of your perception during your exploration of the body will reveal many examples of symmetry of form.

Try pressing hard around the nail bed to relieve toothache

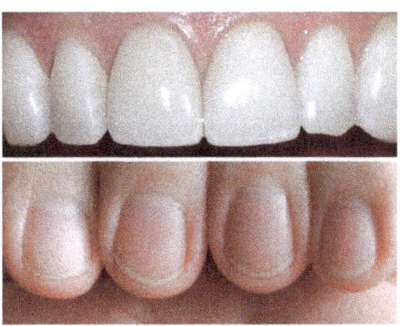

Harmonics

Apart from the use of mathematics and geometry to understand the world, man has always understood that sound has a fundamental expression in nature and the cosmos as a whole. The concept that the universe is ordered in a manner consistent with principles of musical harmony were first expounded by Pythagoras.

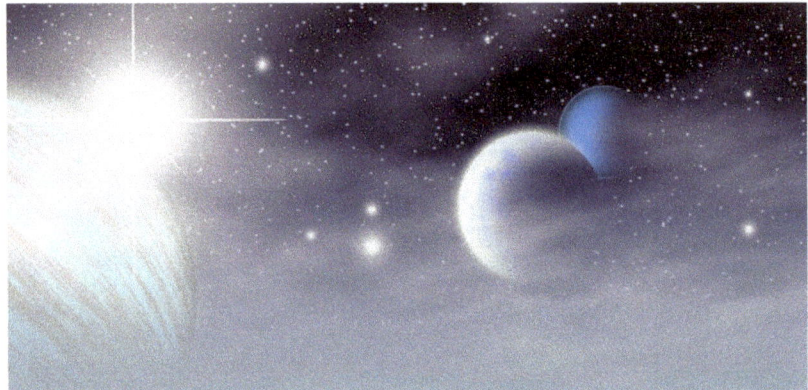

There is geometry in the humming of the strings, there is music in the spacing of the spheres. Pythagoras

When Pythagoras first began experimenting with a single piece of stretched cord (what is now known as a monochord) he made an outstanding discovery. When the cord was halved it sounded the same note but at a higher pitch than the original. He had discovered the ratio 2:1 (the octave). Simply put, if you play a string, then stop the string at half its length, it will sound a note that is exactly an octave higher. Further experimentation with differing lengths of cord exposed different ratios, all producing sounds that were pleasing to the ear. He concluded that harmonic music was produced through exact numerical ratios of whole numbers. From this, he came to believe that the whole universe was musical; that the heavenly spheres produced tones at varying levels as they orbited in their prescribed trajectories across the galaxy. The various proportions within the movements of the planets expressed the music of the spheres—a celestial harmony. Music, Pythagoras believed, was number made audible.

The harmonics of sound provides another way to understand the creation of the correspondences in the body. The human body is a rich tapestry of harmonious, rhythmic, energetic vibrations. Every organ, every cell even, has its own unique frequency beating to the rhythm of Life. In order for the orchestra of the body to be sound, that is to say, well and healthy, each part of the body needs to be free to vibrate otherwise the frequency is compromised and therefore out of tune with the whole.

Cymatics, the study of visible sound and vibration, has shown that varying sound frequencies create and sustain different forms. Humans have always recognised the power of the different vibrations associated with different sounds and their affects on mind, body and spirit. More than this, there is the belief that certain sounds can even restore order to the cosmos. The Navajo believe that Changing Woman, the personification of the Earth and of the natural order of the universe, sings the world into being, thereby maintaining Ho'zho' the beauty and harmony of the universe. The belief that 'word' creates reality.

The earth will be, the mountains will be . . . ,

The earth will be, from ancient times with me there is knowledge of it.

The mountains will be, from ancient times with me there is knowledge of it. . . .

The earth will be, from the very beginning I have thought it. The mountains will be, from the very beginning I have thought it. . . .

The earth will be, from the ancient times I speak it.

The mountains will be, from the ancient times I speak it. . . . The earth will be, the mountains will be, . . .

and so it will be.

(from Navajo, the Beginning of the World Song)

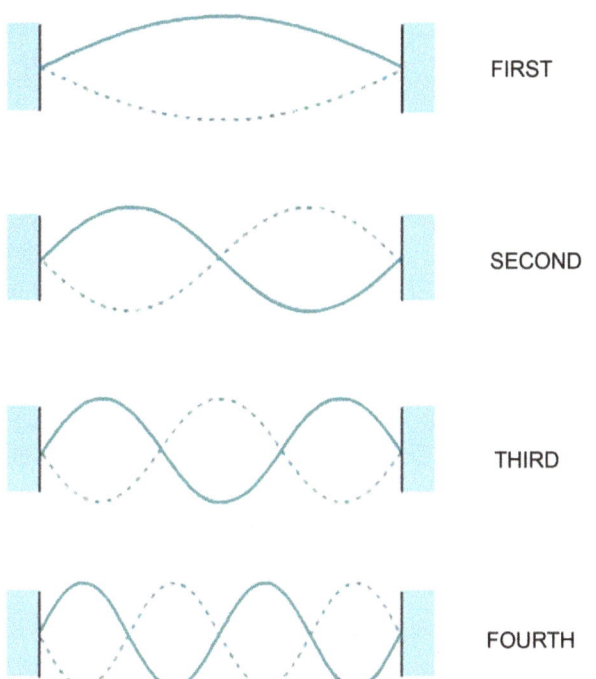

FIRST

SECOND

THIRD

FOURTH

Depending upon where a single stringed musical instrument (a monochord) is stopped different notes or frequencies of sound arise when the string is plucked.

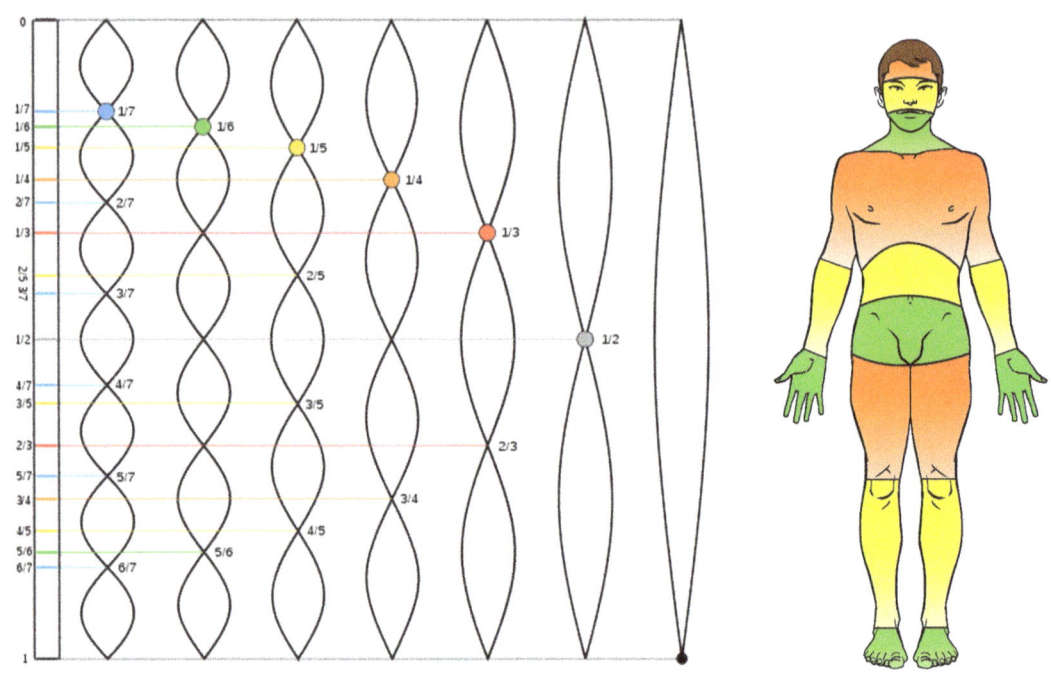

Correspondences in the human body can be thought of as a harmonic relationship of parts.

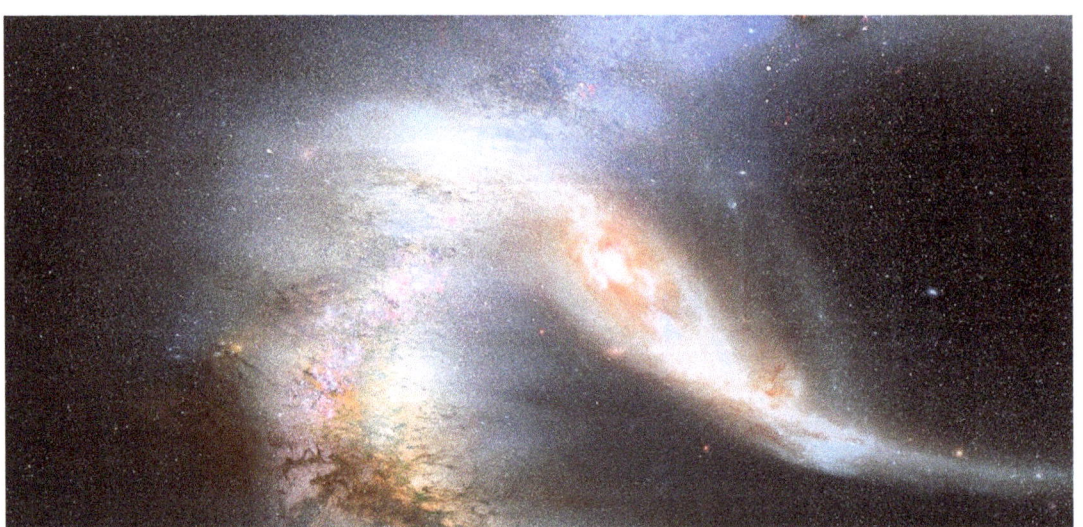

"...for there is music wherever there is harmony, order, or proportion; and thus far we may maintain the music of the spheres".

Thomas Browne

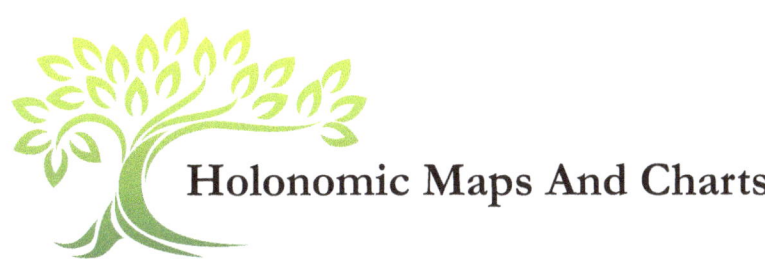

Holonomic Maps And Charts

The Reflex Charts of Holonomic Reflexology

A true cartography of the human being

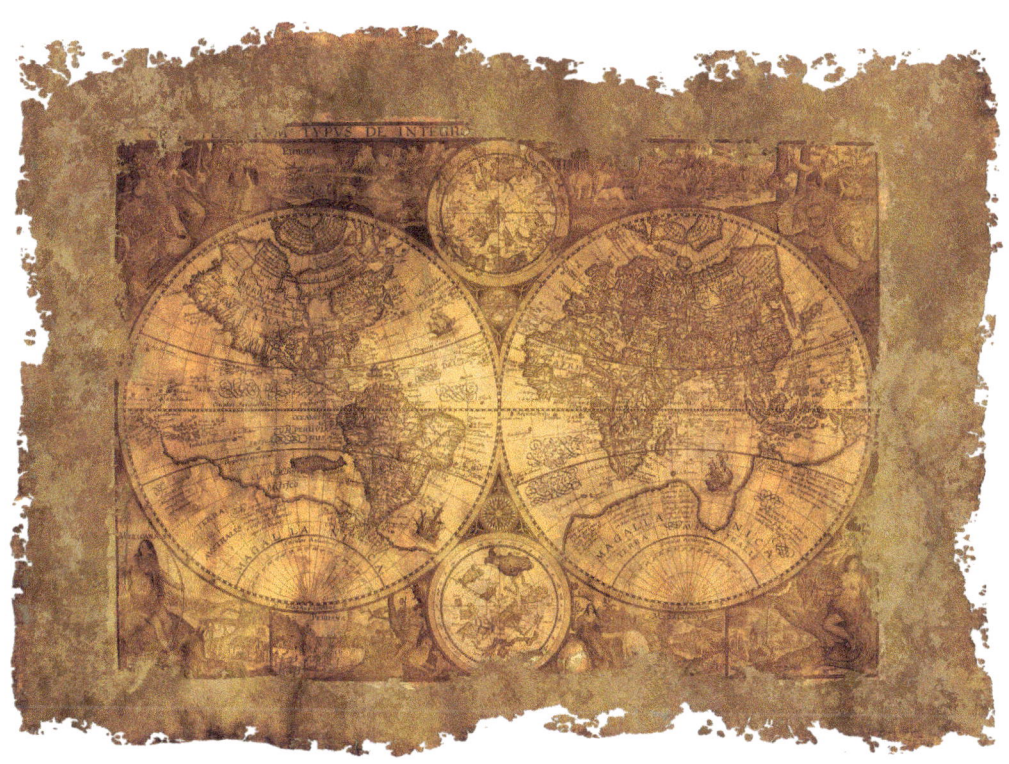

"The map is not the territory"

Count Alfred Korzybski

INVOLUTIONARY CORRESPONDENCES
INTO THE WORLD

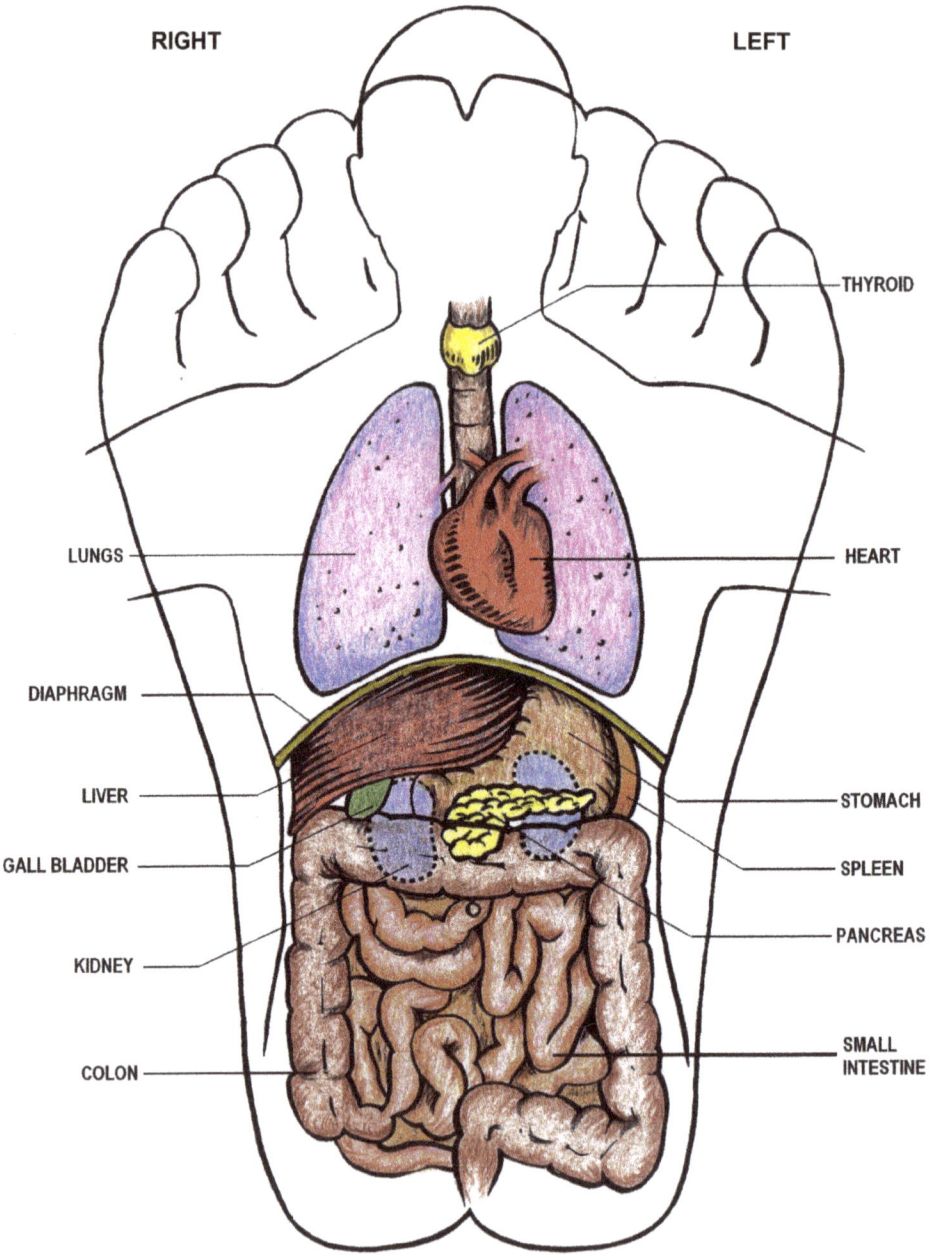

Relative position of body organs on the soles of the feet

THE BODY AND SPINE IN THE FEET
Two classic reflexology charts

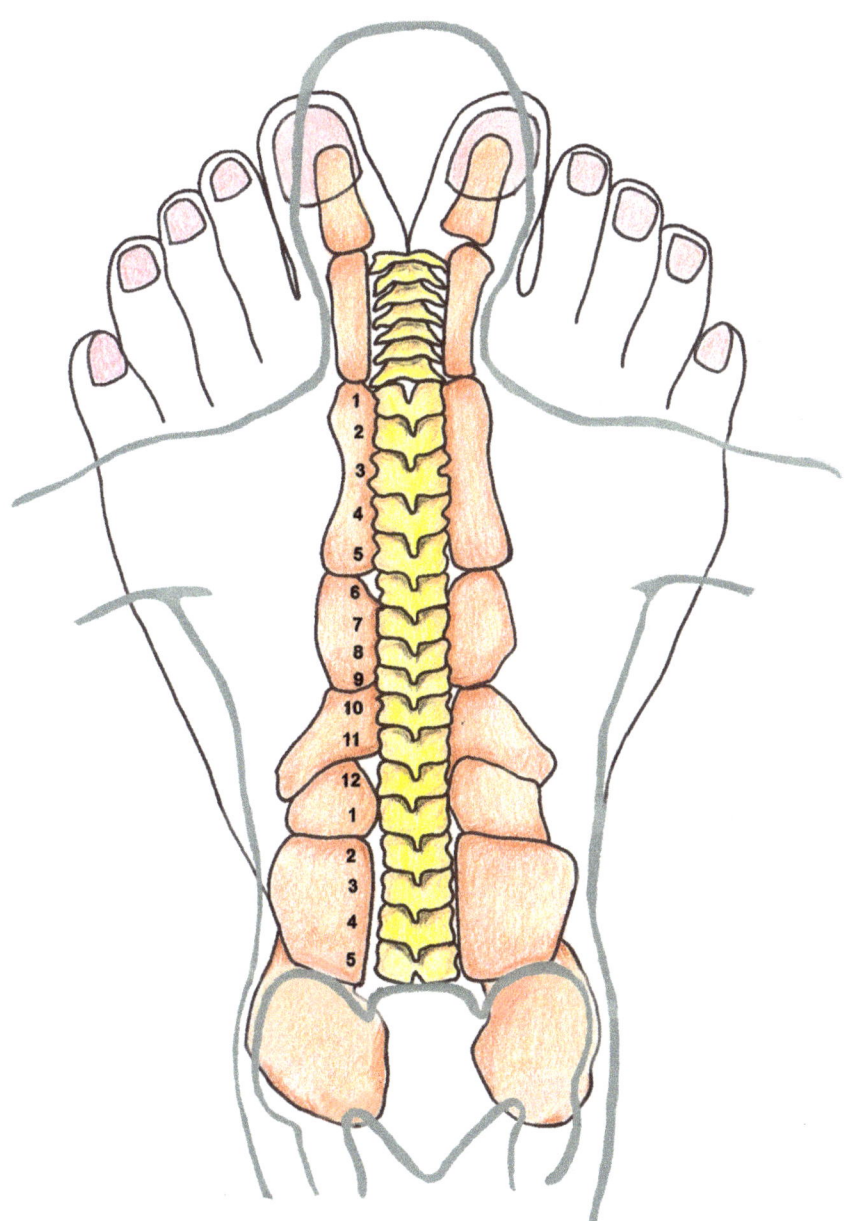

Spinal vertebrae in relation to the bones of the feet

THE ENERGY CENTRES

The chakras, as individual centres of the life energy each possessing a different quality and consciousness, support the functioning of the body and mind.

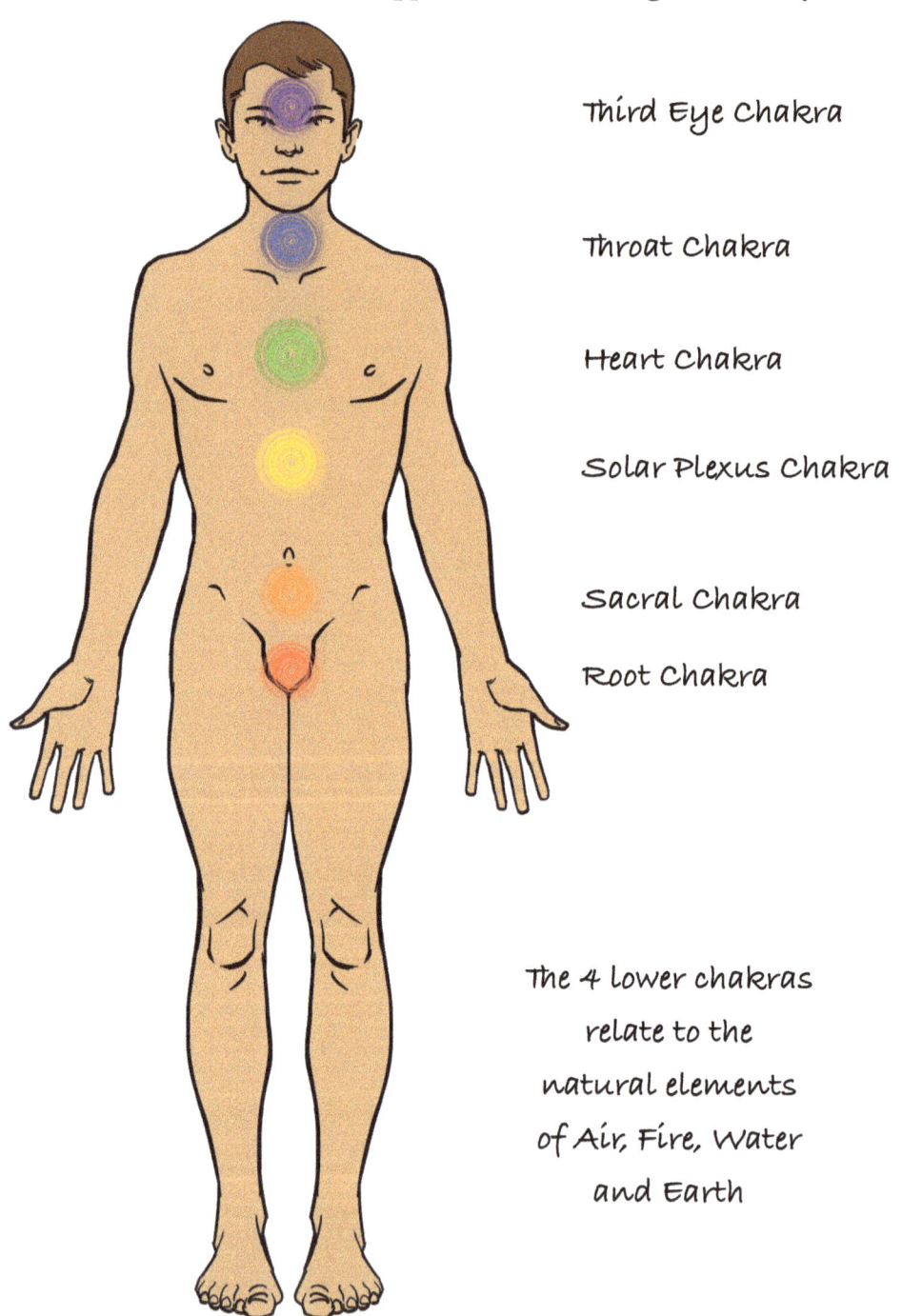

Third Eye Chakra

Throat Chakra

Heart Chakra

Solar Plexus Chakra

Sacral Chakra

Root Chakra

The 4 lower chakras relate to the natural elements of Air, Fire, Water and Earth

LONGITUDINAL ENERGY FLOWS

Life energy currents emanating from the five lower energy centres of the body, create long line currents (or longitudinal zones)

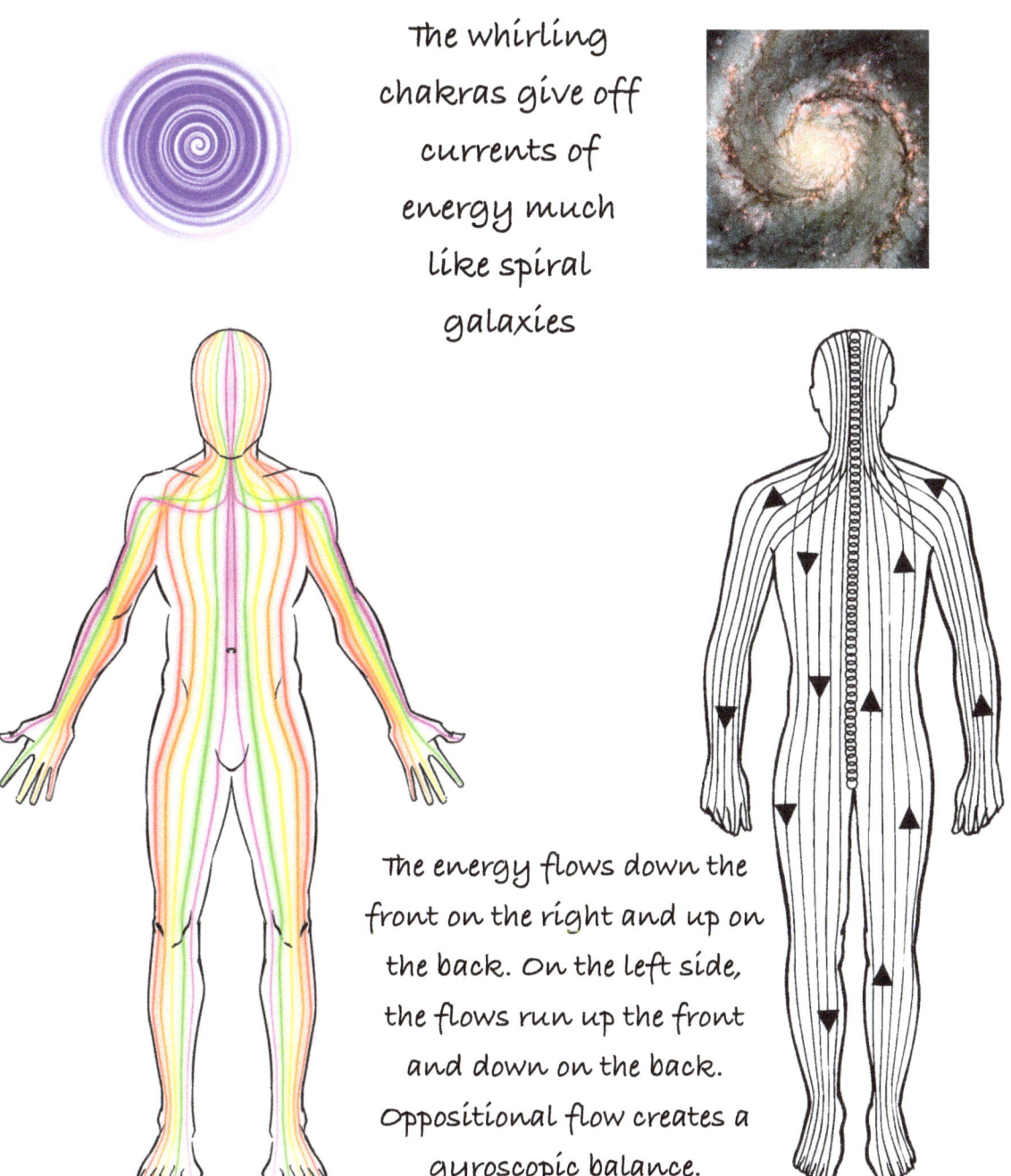

The whirling chakras give off currents of energy much like spiral galaxies

The energy flows down the front on the right and up on the back. On the left side, the flows run up the front and down on the back. Oppositional flow creates a gyroscopic balance.

DR. FITZGERALD'S ORIGINAL ZONE CHARTS

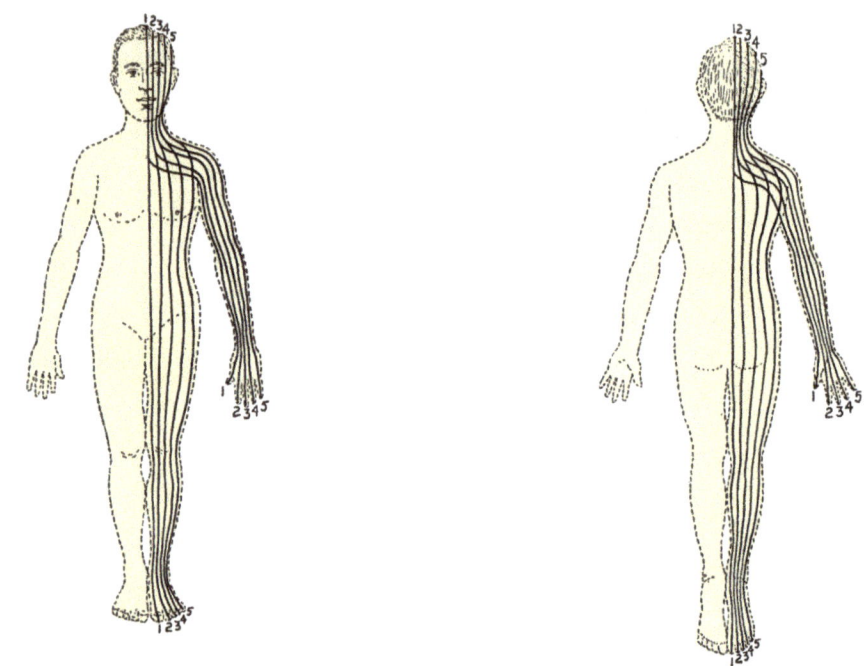

The Zones re-interpreted as Energy Flows

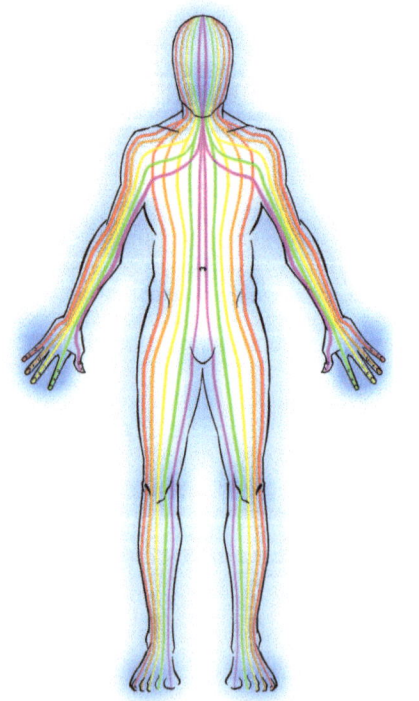
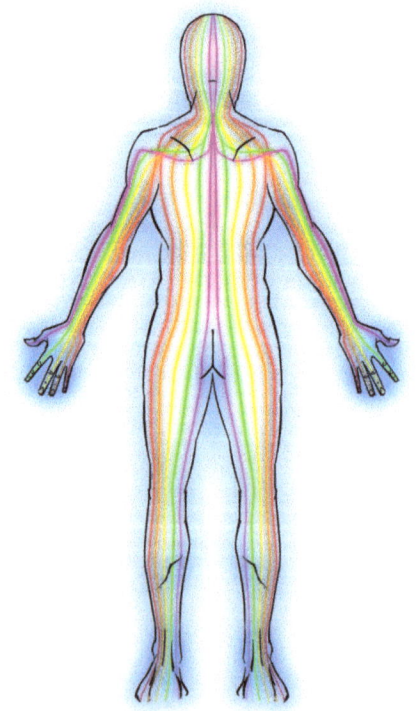

BODY ZONES
The body divided into 9 zones

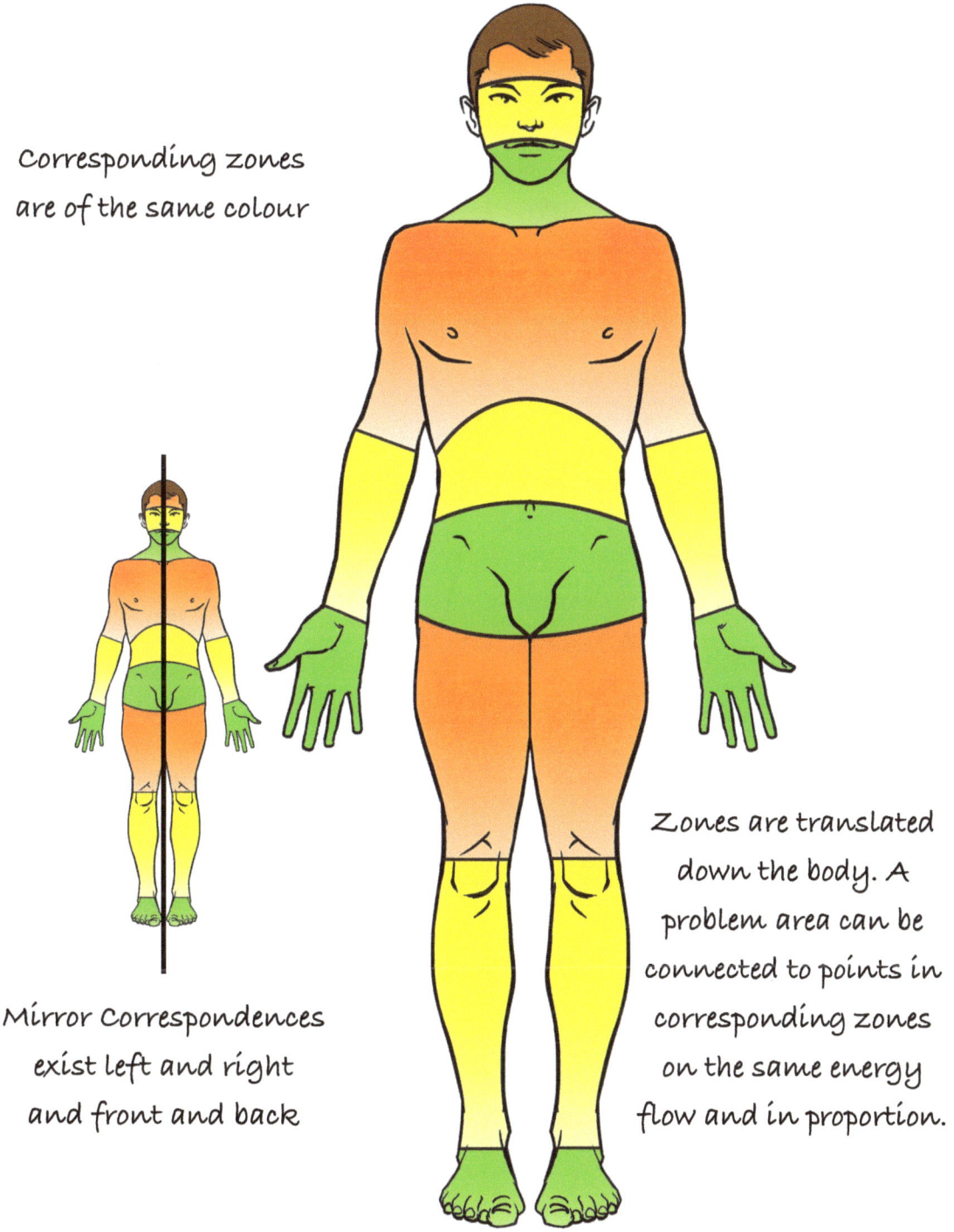

Corresponding zones are of the same colour

Mirror Correspondences exist left and right and front and back

Zones are translated down the body. A problem area can be connected to points in corresponding zones on the same energy flow and in proportion.

VERTICAL ZONES OF HANDS AND FEET

The body zones are also reflected in the hands and feet giving rise to more correspondences such as the heel of the foot and the heel of the hand

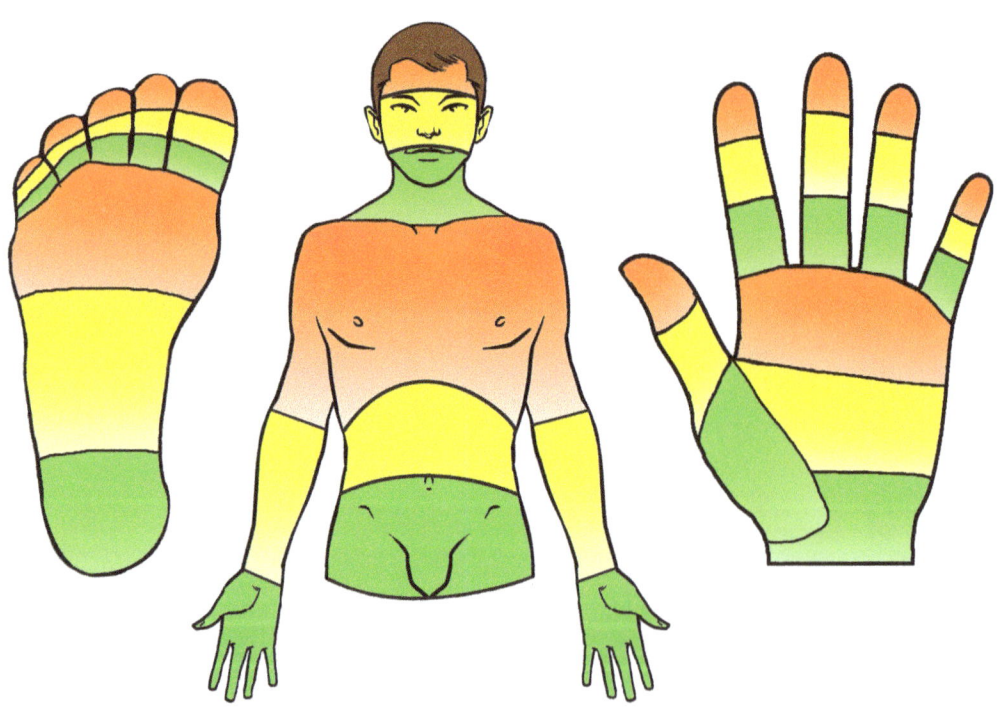

Acute conditions may be successfully treated from the hand reflexes whereas more chronic conditions may respond better to areas on the feet.

HORIZONTAL ZONES OF HANDS AND FEET

The body divided into 9 different zones based upon a horizontal orientation of the hands and feet ot the body.

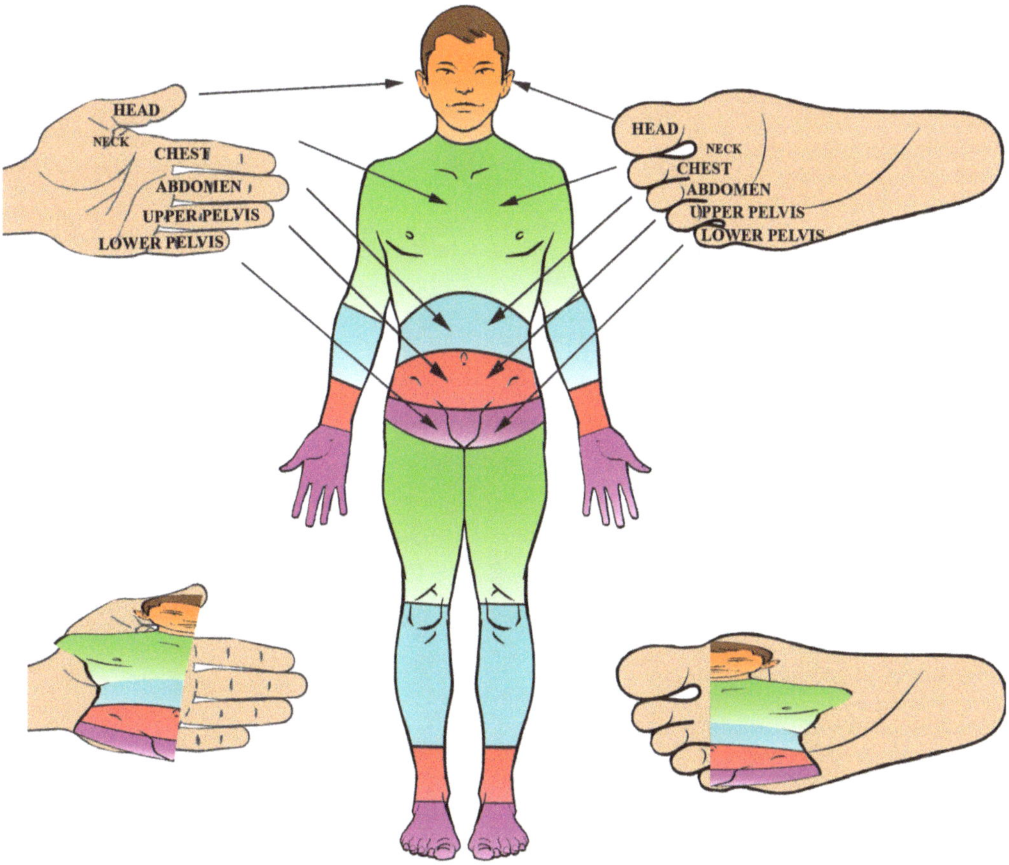

The body can be divided into any number of harmonics all showing potential correspondences

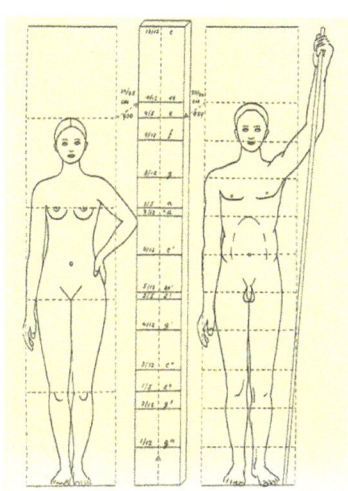

GEOMETRIC CORRESPONDENCES

This chart is derived from Robert Fludd's work on the monochord, a harmonic perspective on the Universe which shows man as microcosm in the macrocosm.

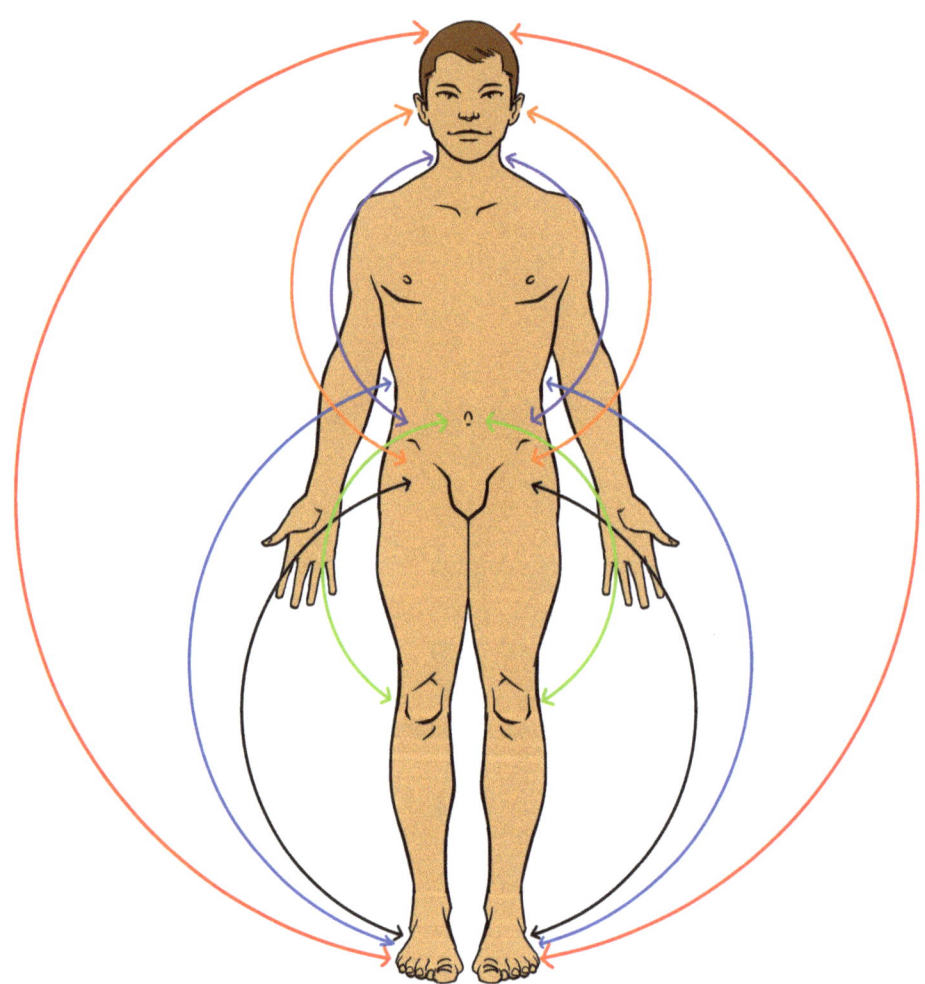

"This, is the world monochord, with its proportions, harmonies and intervals of its extra-mundane movement accurately spaced as herein depicted".

Musica Mundane - Robert Fludd

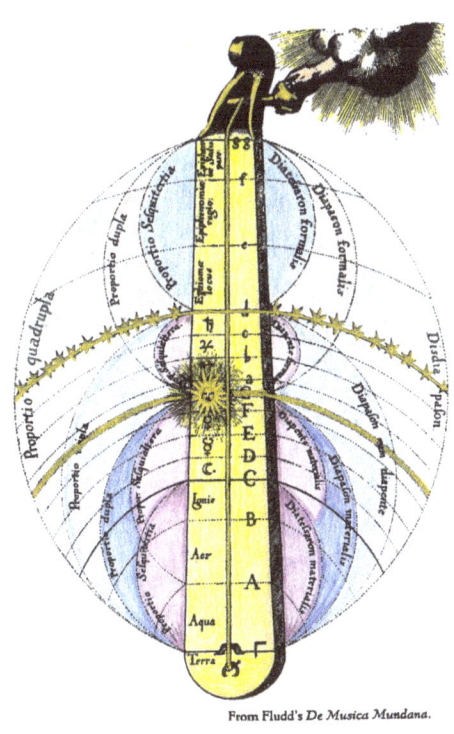

From Fludd's *De Musica Mundana*.

When the concept of the monochord is applied to the human body correspondences appear

SIGNIFICANT CORRESPONDENCES

Ankle/Hip

Sacro-iliac joints/Condyles of the skull

Mastoid bone/Ilium

Knees/Navel

Ears/Hip joint

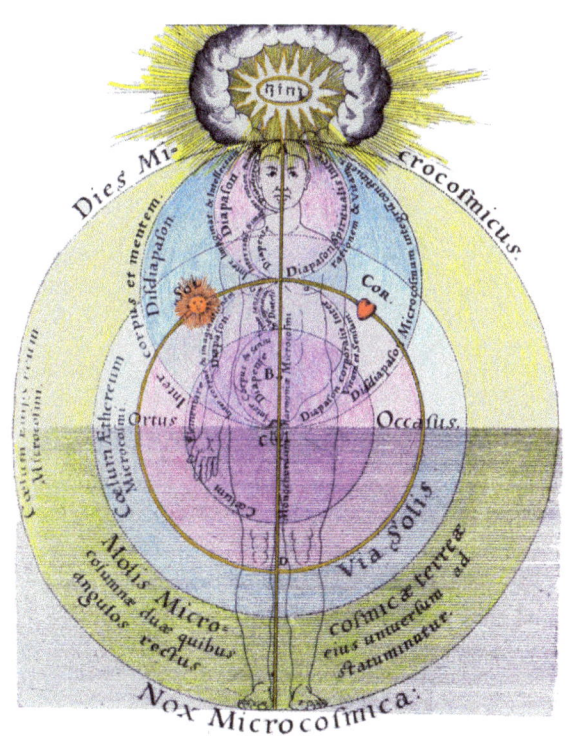

ASTROLOGICAL CORRESPONDENCES

The body is woven in the womb from the 4 natural elements of Air, Fire, Water and Earth

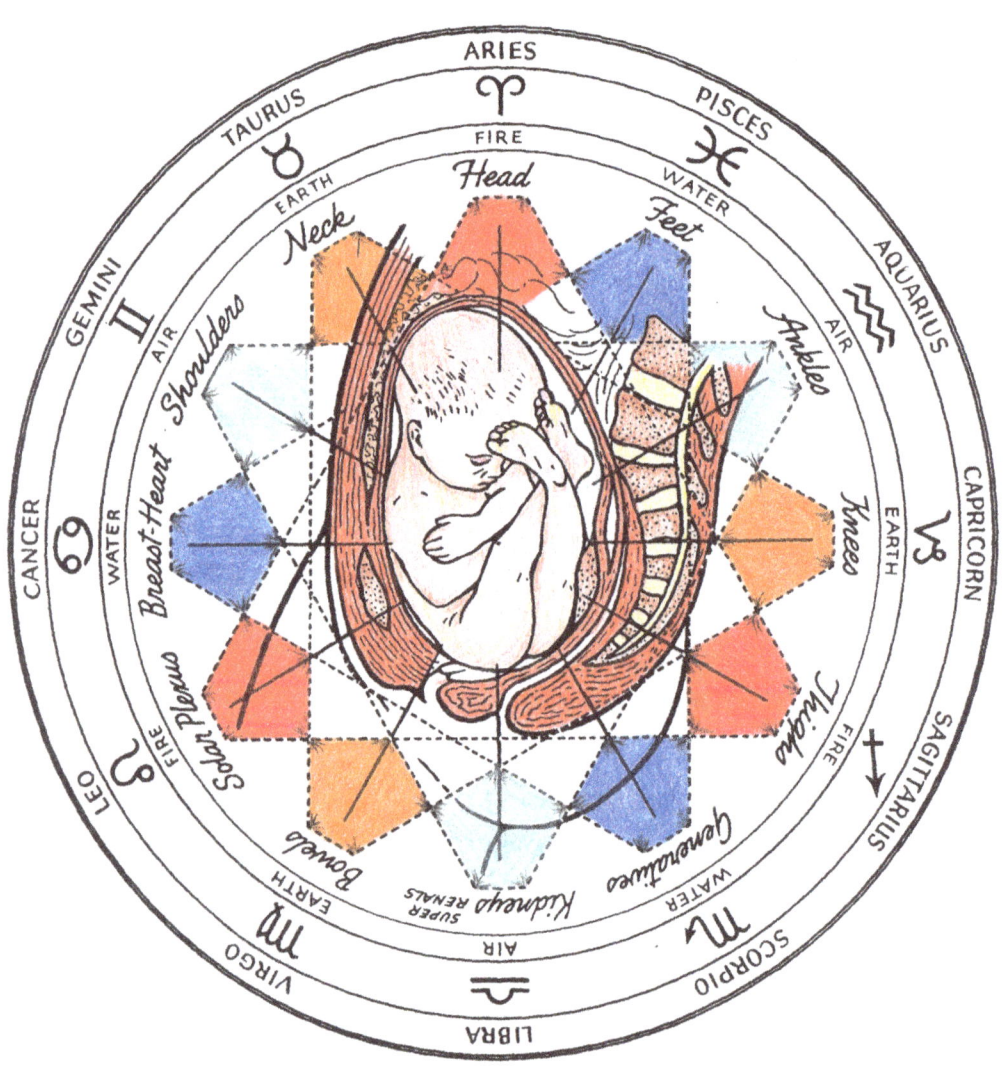

The previous chart is a more modern interpretation of an ancient chart on the form of man shown below

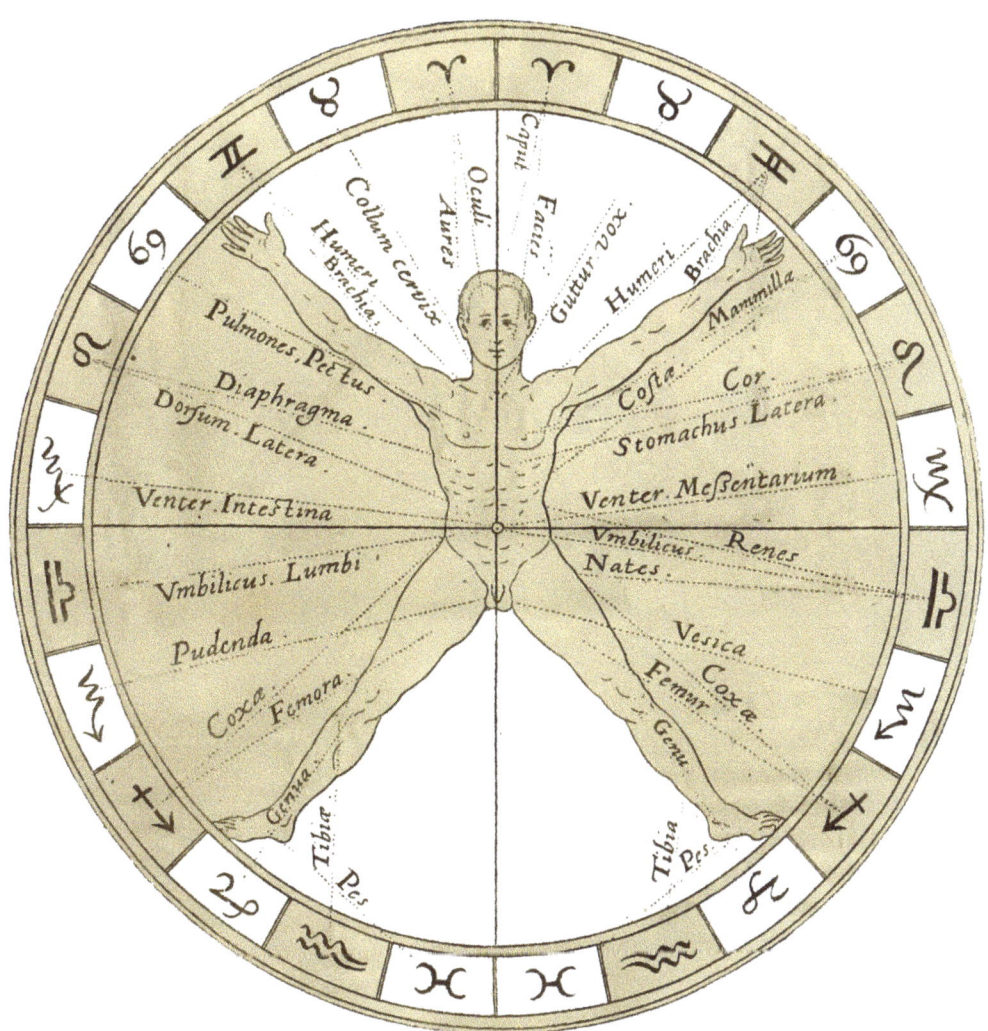

Zodiac Man—Robert Fludd

Our entry into the world follows the order of the Zodiac

CONSCIOUSNESS IN THE BODY

This chart illustrates how the cranium, representing consciousness, pervades and influences the body

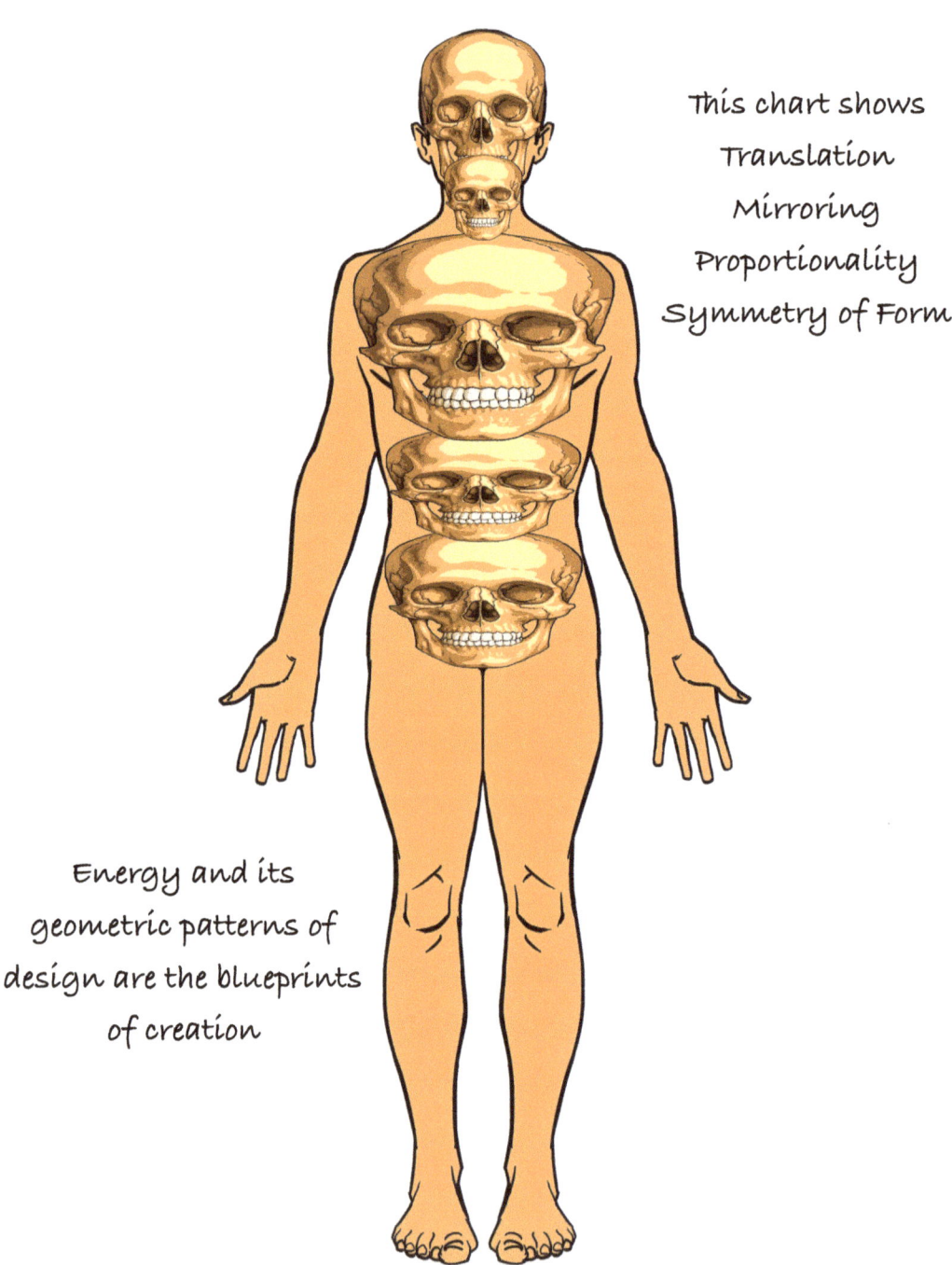

The head is translated into each cavity of the body, throat, chest, upper abdomen and pelvis

Some of the most significant correspondences are to found between the head and the pelvis

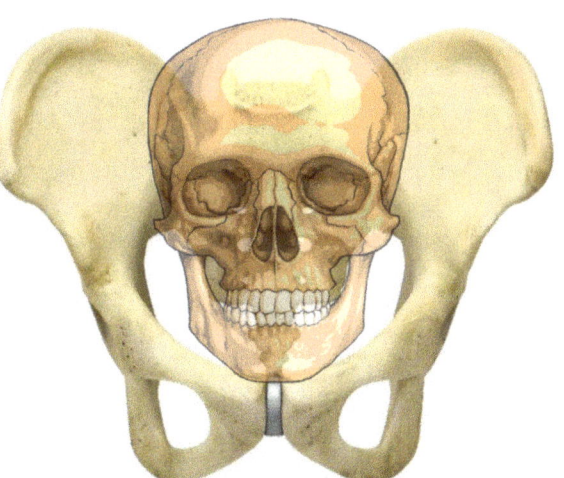

SIGNIFICANT REFLEXES

Eyes/Liver and Stomach/Ovaries

Lower Jaw/Clavicle/Respiratory Diaphragm/Pubic Bone

CRANIAL PELVIC REFLEXES

TMJ/Hip joint

Jaw/Symphysis pubis

Parietal bone/Innominate bone

Occipital base/Sacral base

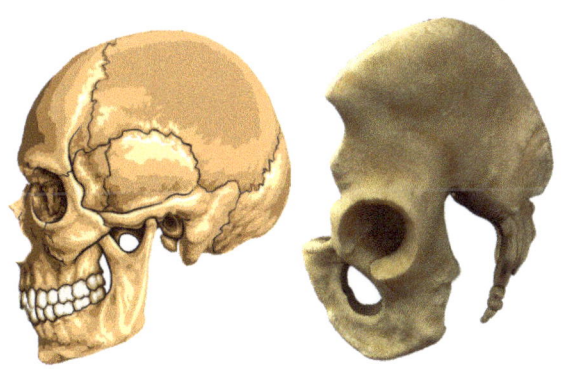

SPINAL CORRESPONDENCES

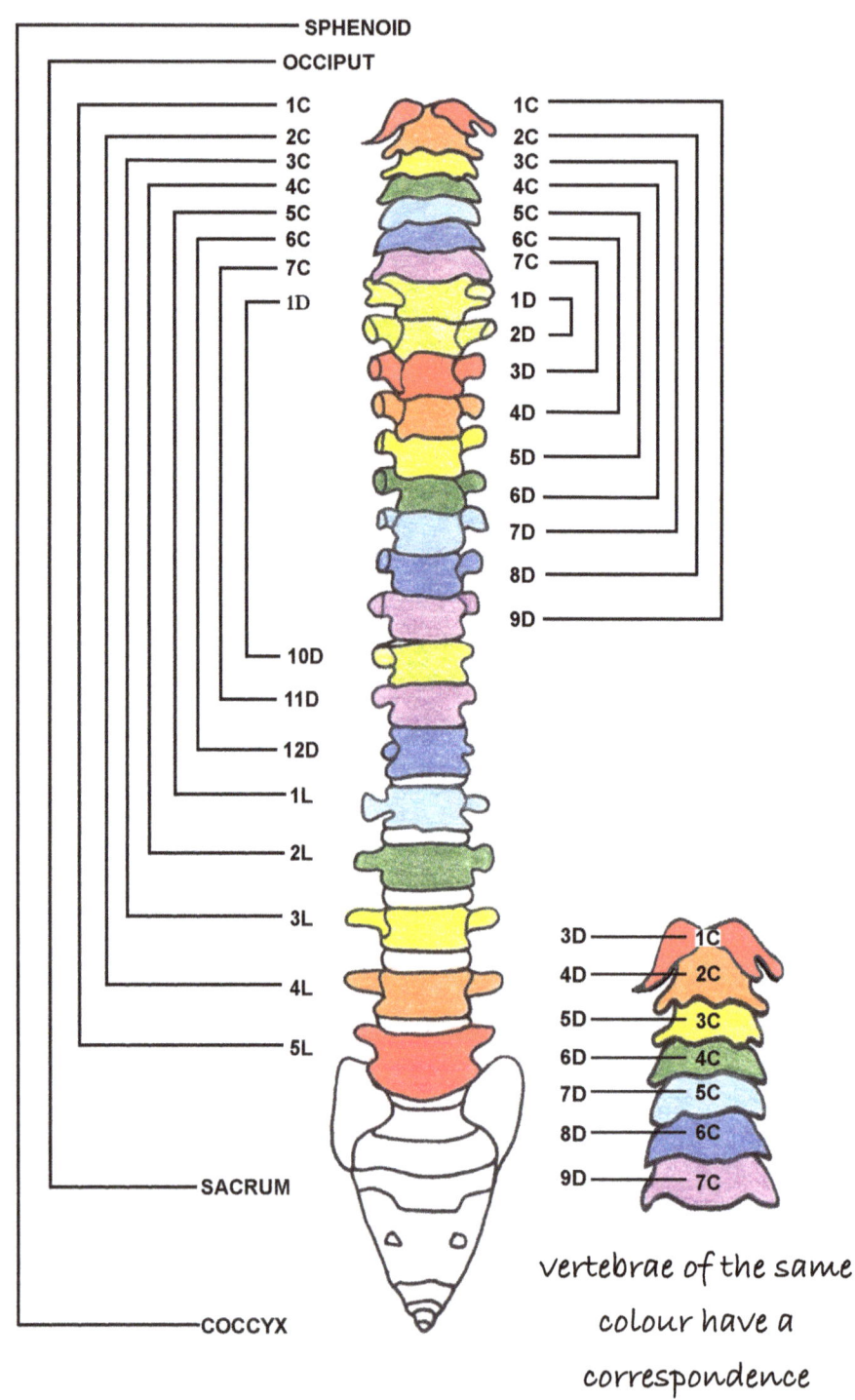

vertebrae of the same colour have a correspondence

6 POINTED STAR

Birth and Re-birth

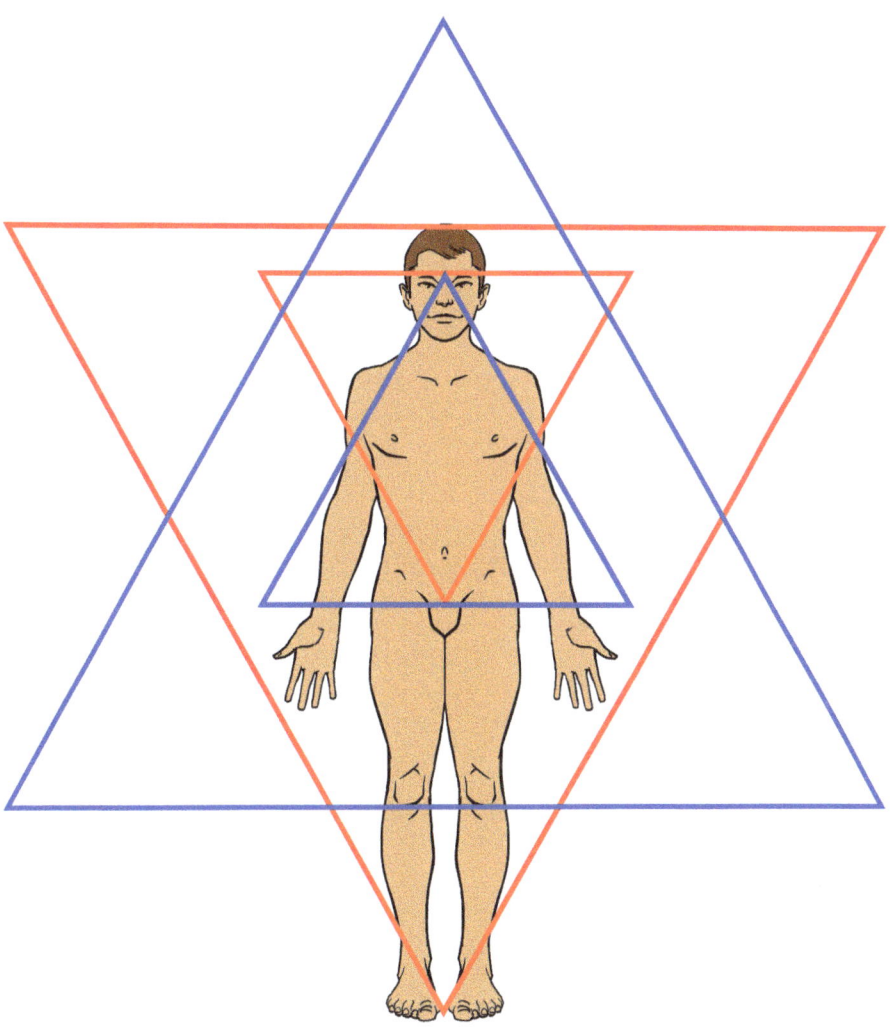

The 6 pointed star can be envisioned on the body giving rise to a special correspondence between the third eye and the pubis

It can also exist as a larger star in the energy field around the body

EVOLUTIONARY CORRESPONDENCES
BACK TO SOURCE

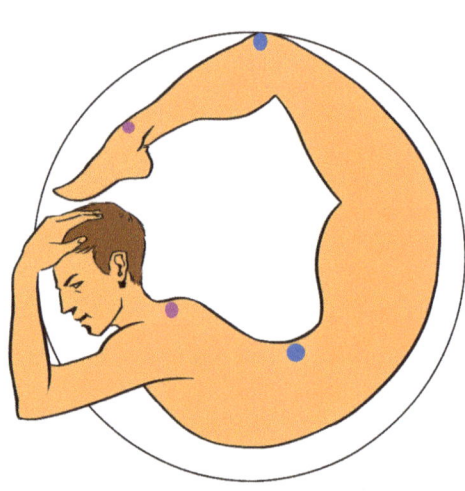

Various interpretations of a chart (right) originally created by Max Heindel

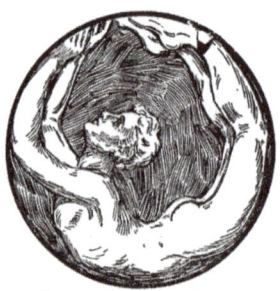

BENT OUTWARDS
AS CELESTIAL SPHERES
CONSCIOUSNESS IN THE CENTER

The patella relates to L2/L3 on the back and the top of the ankle to the brachial plexus. The spine has correspondences on the top of the foot and front of the leg

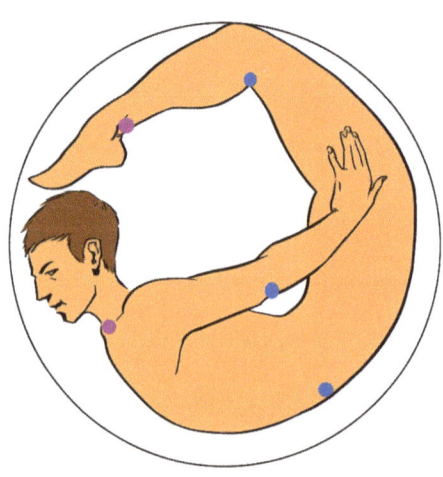

The body in this evolutionary bow position is the exact opposite of the involutionary foetal position

Inside of knee relates to inside elbow and umbilicus. The achilles tendon relates to the throat

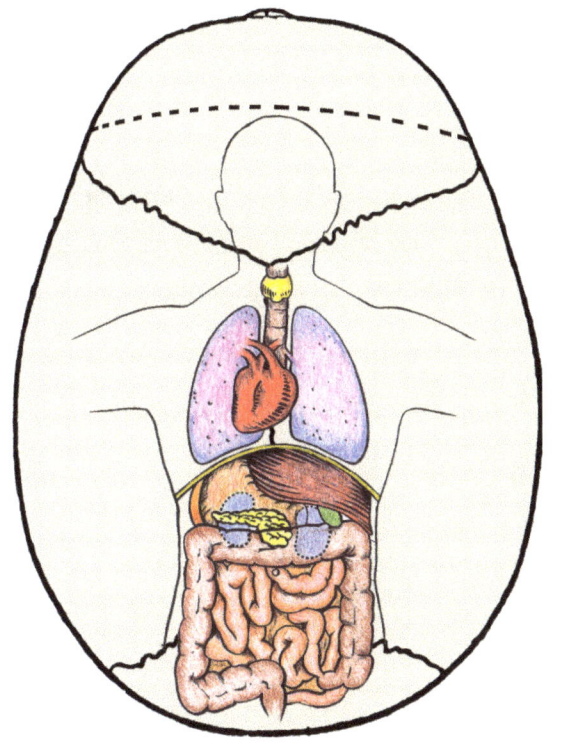

Evolutionary Reflexes on the top of the head

The chart shows organ reflexes on the top of the head

Spinal reflexes on the feet align along the sagittal suture on the top of the head.

The cervical spine starts at the anterior fontanel and progresses back to the posterior fontanel

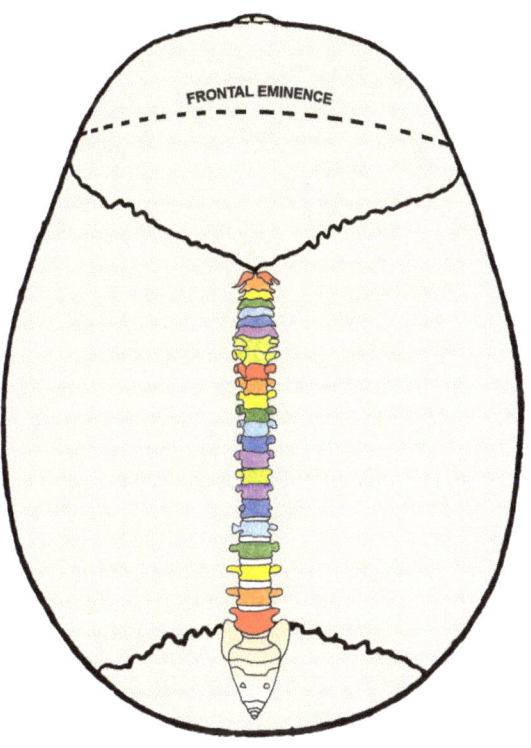

THE BODY IN CONSCIOUSNESS

The body reflected in the head

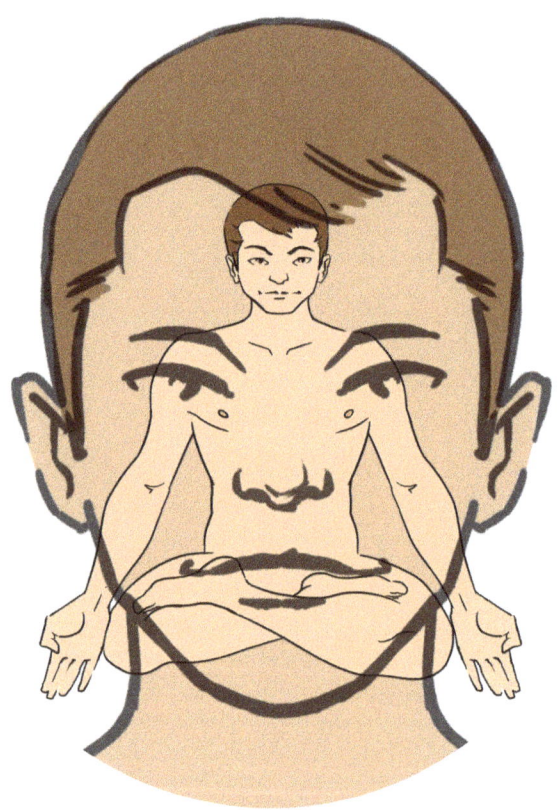

Discolouration, tension and skin disruptions can indicate problems in related body part and can aid diagnosis

The body reflected in the ear

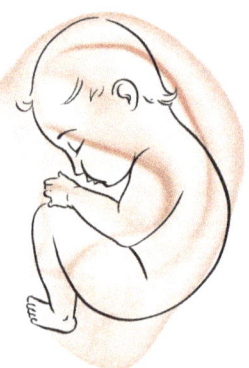

The buttocks reflect the fleshy lobe of the ear whilst the head is reflected in the pinna of the upper ear. The ear canal can be seen as a correspondence to the umbilicus

SIGNIFICANT CORRESPONDENCES

Eyes / Shoulder sockets

Mouth / Generative Organs

Upper jaw / Digestive organs

5 POINTED STAR
Endless Regeneration

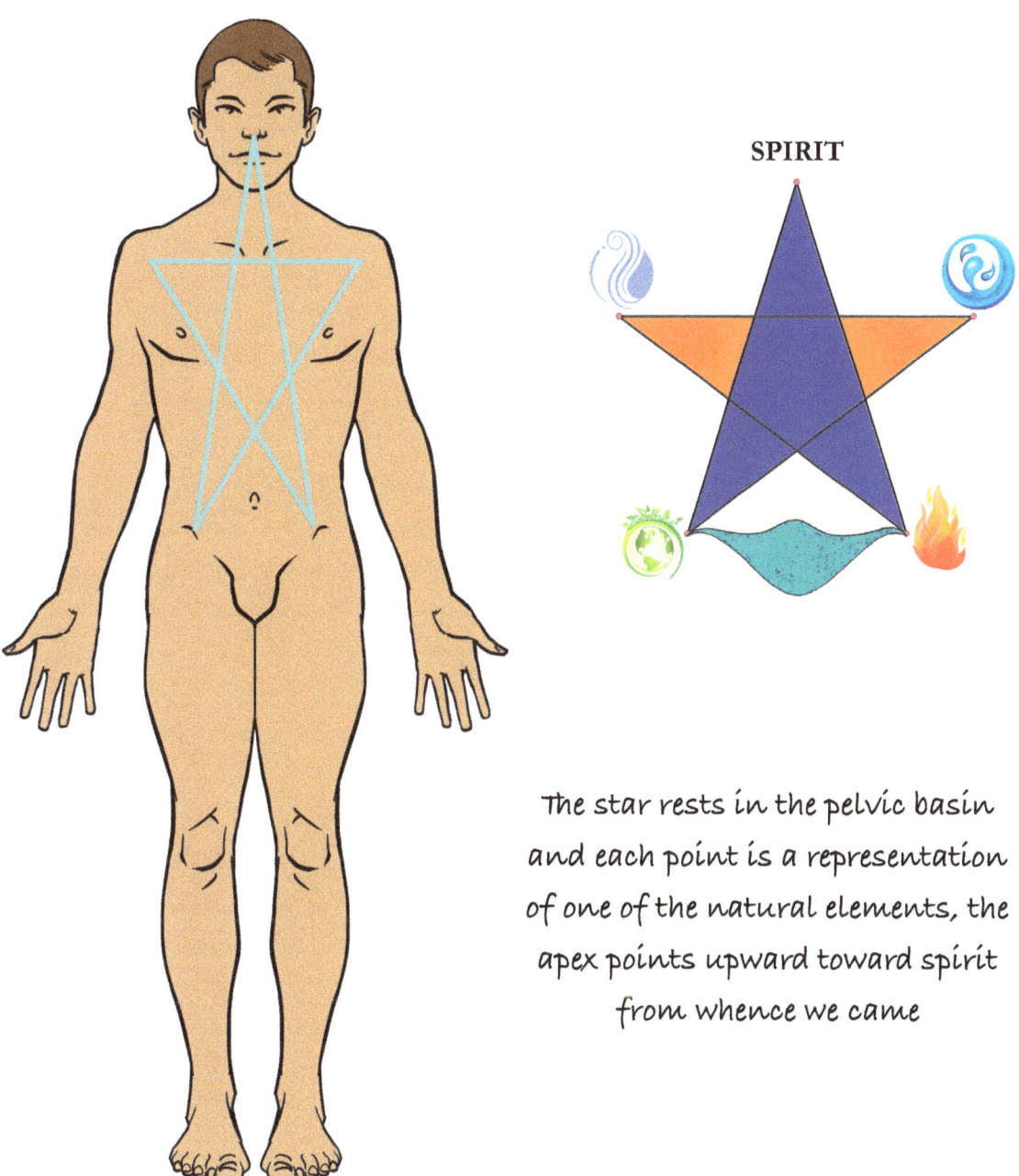

The star rests in the pelvic basin and each point is a representation of one of the natural elements, the apex points upward toward spirit from whence we came

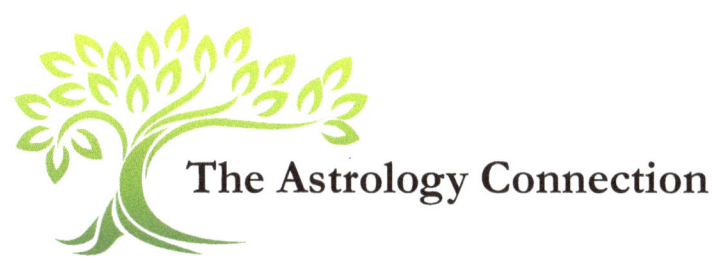

The Astrology Connection

"Whatever is Below is like unto that which is Above, and whatever is Above is like unto that which is Below, to accomplish the miracle of the One".

Hermes Trismegistus

The night sky has been a source of wonder since mankind first walked the Earth. The first constellations, as we now know them, were recognised and named, in Mesopotamia, around 3000BC. However, the Babylonians are often considered to be the first true astronomers. It is they who introduced the concept of the Zodiac realising that the sequence of the constellations, as they move across the sky, can serve as a yardstick of celestial time when divided into twelve equal segments. They selected twelve constellations to represent each of the segments and each constellation came to be associated with a specific god, which acknowledged and paid homage to a Divine influence.

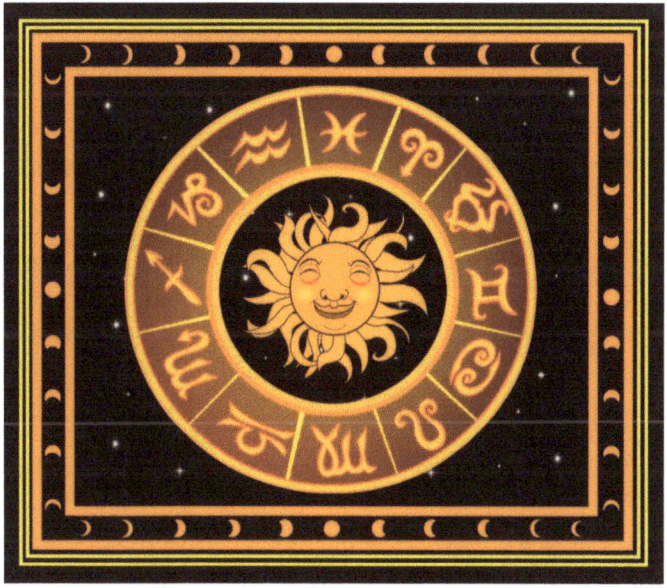

"One of the divine principles that work in nature—the human being is the result of the influences of the stars in other words, of the creating beings".

Paracelsus

There has long been an awareness that the movement of the celestial constellations around the heavens and the planets of our own solar system have effects on, and consequences for, life on Earth.

Originally, Astrology was used for predicting such things as the weather, guiding decision and policy making and foretelling the coming of major events. One such event, the first plague epidemic in Europe in 1348, was believed by the then Pope's physician, Guy de Ghauliac, to have been caused by a conjunction of Saturn, Mars and Jupiter.

At the end of the late 1500s physicians across Europe were actually required by law to calculate the position of the moon, our nearest planet, before carrying out complicated medical procedures, especially those involving surgery. In the time before the advent of medicines, as we now know them, right up to the 17th century, Astrology continued to be used as a major tool in the diagnosis of any number of aches, pains and illnesses.

The constellations and the planets of our solar system exert a large field of influence on us. The sun is the most obvious influence and our moon is also well known for its effects here on Earth. The influence of the moon on our health is recognised by today's medical practitioners. It has been found that the cycles of the moon influence sleep patterns, mental conditions and fertility, (women are generally more fertile in the dark of the moon just before the new moon is visible).

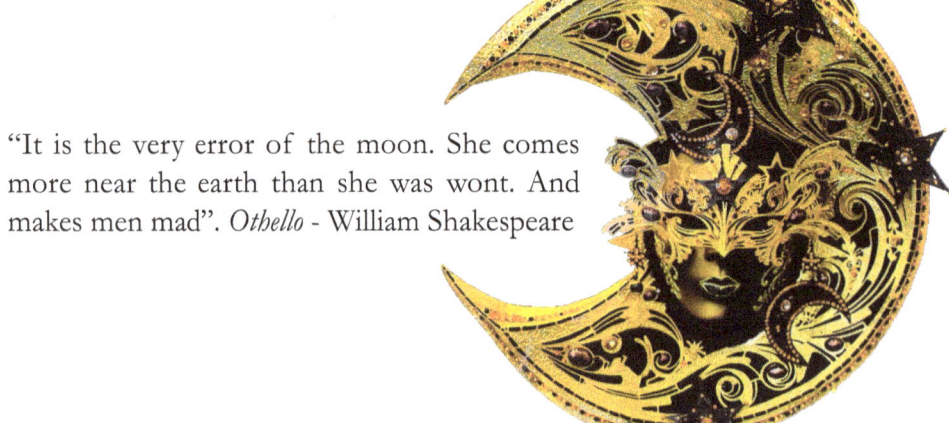

"It is the very error of the moon. She comes more near the earth than she was wont. And makes men mad". *Othello* - William Shakespeare

Whilst the life energy acts as a blueprint for the human body, these celestial bodies influence and inform our physiological functioning through their emanations which directly affect our life energy.

Zodiac is a Greek word meaning "circle of animals" and each segment of the circle, which represents a part of the year, was given the name of an animal or, in a few cases, types of people or objects.

20 March to 20 April - Aries—the Ram

21 April to 20 May - Taurus—the Bull

21 May to 20 June - Gemini—the Twins

21 June to 22 July - Cancer—the Crab

23 July to 22 Aug - Leo—the Lion

23 August to 22 September - Virgo—the Maiden

23 September to 22 October - Libra—the Scales

23 October to 21 November - Scorpio—the Scorpion

22 November to 21 December - Sagittarius—the Centaur

22 December to 19 January - Capricorn—the Goat

20 January to 18 February - Aquarius—the Waterbearer

19 February to 20 March - Pisces—the Fishes

On the 20th of March of each year the Sun moves back into the sign of Aries again

> "A physician without a knowledge of Astrology has no right to call himself a physician".
>
> Hippocrates

Astrology has taken on a somewhat different colouration in the modern world. Today, most people understand Astrology as a system that provides insight into the character and psychology of an individual, as the astrological sign we are born under has an influence on our temperament. It is still perhaps most universally used as a predictive tool, though for most part this is limited to perusing a daily horoscope. The emphasis on the medical aspect of Astrology has diminished. Each sign of the Zodiac has its own characteristics, some of which can be surmised from their name. Thus, those born under the sign of Capricorn, the goat, 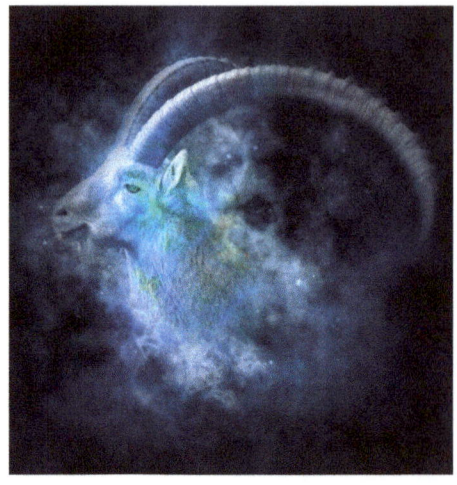 can be surefooted and steadfast, like to get to the top, so can be ambitious and are normally even tempered. However, you can expect a hefty butt from those horns when they are riled. Those born under the sign of Cancer, on the other hand, can be bad tempered and crabby, which is usually just a defence against the vulnerability of that soft underside and they may have a tendency to hold onto things with those giant claws.

These are just light hearted and superficial descriptions, but they make the point. It is not the purpose of this book to go into the details of Astrology, which is a study in its own right.

> "All qualities, energies and forces of the planets are latent within us, like in a magic Sesame Cave, and we decide what jewels we will use out of Life's Treasures every day, every hour and with every thought. How rich we are and know it not!".
> *Alchemical Astrology* - Dr. Randolph Stone

The first sign of the Zodiac begins in March at the time of the Spring equinox, a nodal point, when the day and the night are of equal length in the Northern hemisphere. This equinox signals a time of new birth after the winter months.

For the purposes of Holonomic Reflexology, it is useful to know the Zodiac signs as each sign relates to a part of the human body (see p. 62/3). To understand how this relationship was created we need to consider the birth process. As the baby emerges from the womb the head appears first and so relates to the first sign of the Zodiac, which is Aries. The next part to emerge is the neck, which relates to Taurus, the sign of the Zodiac which follows Aries. The sequence of the remaining signs follows the order of the parts of the body as they emerge into the world. The shoulders relate to Gemini. Once the shoulders emerge the chest follows (Cancer) then the solar plexus (Leo), and the bowels (Virgo). The kidneys come next (Libra), then the pelvis and the genital region (Scorpio), followed by the thighs (Sagittarius). Next come the knees (Capricorn), the ankles (Aquarius) and finally the feet (Pisces).

Traditional Astrology maintains that as the sun enters each sign of the Zodiac, its influence is modulated by the emanations of that particular constellation. The Zodiacal sign that the sun is in at the moment of our birth indicates the most dominant astrological influence in our life and has a profound affect on aspects of our constitution. Our constitution is complex. It is affected by ancestral influences, foetal nutrition and environment and, most significantly, the date of our birth. Our basic constitution determines whether we are weak or strong, prone to illness and either slow or quick to recover.

Each sign of the Zodiac falls under the influence of one of four elements. The relationship of each sign of the Zodiac to a particular element gives rise to a unique set of correspondences (see p. 79). Returning to the ancient world for a moment, we know that things were more simple then. Instead of the 118 (as of 2016) elements of our modern periodic table of elements, our ancestors defined the makeup of the world by only four, which were perceivable by their five senses. These elements were Air, Fire, Water and Earth and so each sign of the Zodiac was assigned to one of these four.

The body is woven in the womb from the 4 natural elements

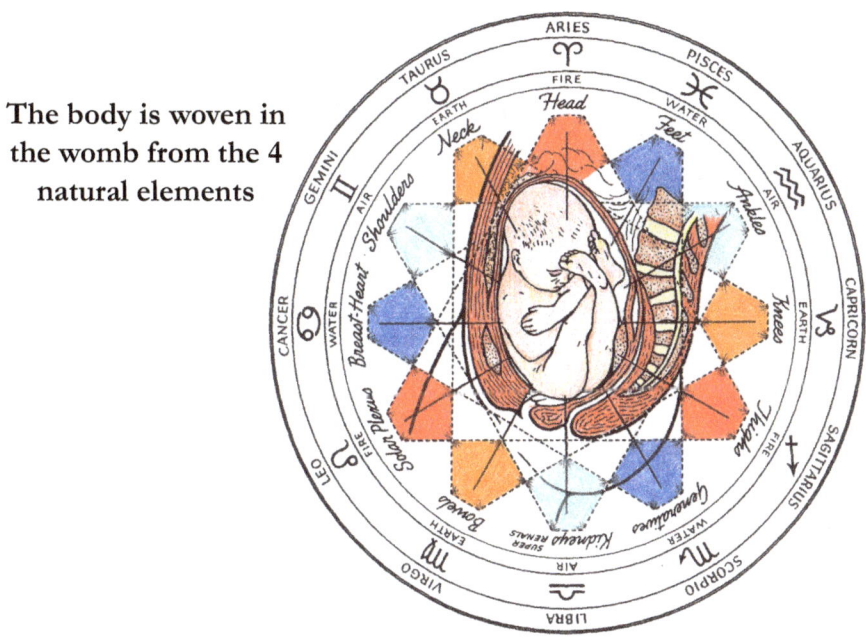

Just like the movements of the constellations and the planets in the heavens and the changing of the seasons, these natural elements also followed cyclic changes. Thus Aries, the first sign of the Zodiac relates to the element of Fire. Taurus follows, which relates to the Earth element, then Gemini, which relates to the Air element and then the sign of Cancer, which relates to the Water element. This elemental order of Fire, Earth, Air and Water then cycles through the rest of the year (see p. 63).

> "We are born at a given moment, in a given place and, like vintage years of wine, we have the qualities of the year and of the season of which we are born. Astrology does not lay claim to anything more".
> Carl Jung

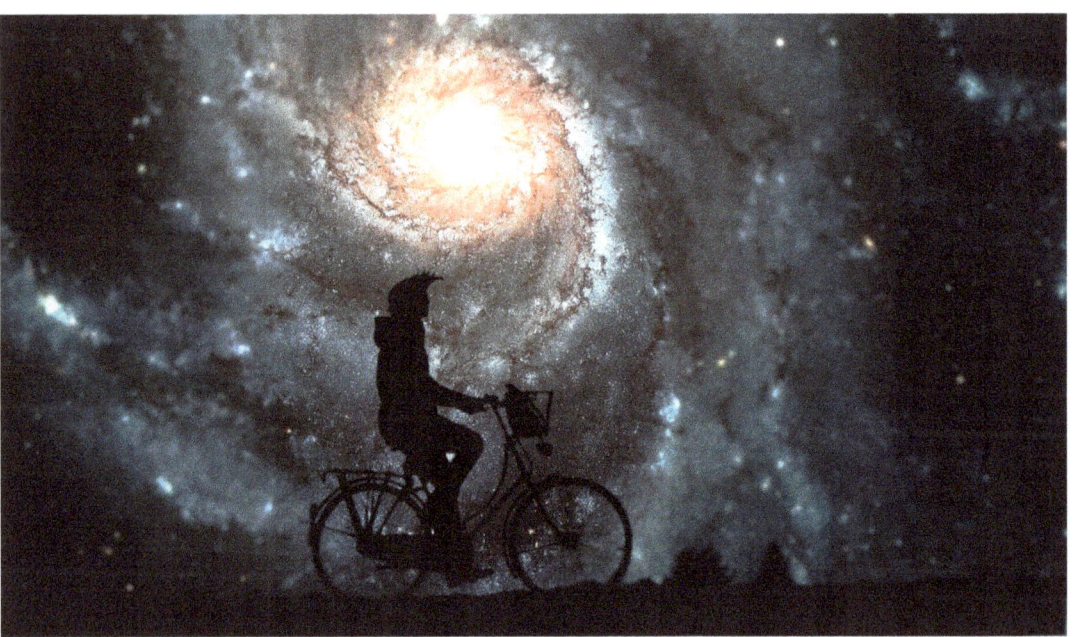

"Living here on Earth, we breathe the rhythms of a universe that extends infinitely above us".

Daisaku Ikeda

Astrological Sign, Element & Body Correspondences

FIRE ELEMENT SIGNS

Aries

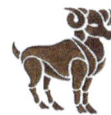 Head/Eyes

Leo

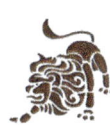 Solar Plexus

Sagittarius

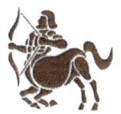 Thighs

EARTH ELEMENT SIGNS

Taurus

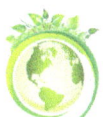 Neck

Virgo

 Bowels

Capricorn

 Knees

AIR ELEMENT SIGNS

Gemini

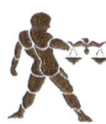 Shoulders

Libra

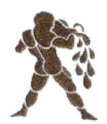 Kidneys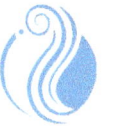

Aquarius

Ankles

WATER ELEMENT SIGNS

Cancer

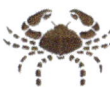 Breast

Scorpio

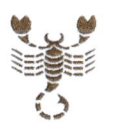 Genitals

Pisces

 Feet

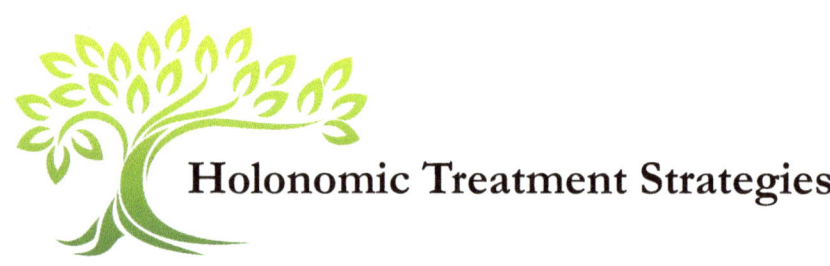

Holonomic Treatment Strategies

Holonomic Reflexology - Summary

- draws on both ancient understandings and principles of life as well as acknowledging and using modern scientific models.

- acknowledges the holistic nature of each of us; that we are indeed the sum of our parts and that when one part is out of tune with the rest it can frequently lead to a globalisation that can result in substantial health problems.

- understands that everything is energy and that robust good health is dependent on the free flow of this life energy throughout the whole being. In other words everything is vibrating and flowing within a unified field. Everything is in relationship with every other part; everything is in direct communication.

- views all correspondences and reflexes in the human being as being a manifestation of God Geometrising.

- uses the multitude of correspondence and reflexes that are present all over the body and which were explored in Dr. Stone's writings on the complete healing system that he called Polarity Therapy.

- views the therapist and client as a conjoint system that behaves as a complex adaptive system.

- perceives human beings as complex and multi-faceted. The maps and charts in Holonomic Reflexology emerge from a range of different perspectives upon human life.

- acknowledges that there is much more to life than just the mundane, that there is a spiritual and sacred dimension to life that is a significant force in relation to health and well-being.

Correspondences and Reflexes

In Holonomic reflexology we do not just work with reflexes but with areas of *correspondence* in the human body.

A correspondence can be defined as any area that has an effect on another area. Correspondences are areas of harmonic resonance.

A reflex can be defined as a point along a current of energy that, when activated, has an effect on other points along that same current of energy.

All reflexes can be defined as a correspondence but not all correspondences are reflexes. Some correspondences are not along the same energy current (or in the same zone) but are in other areas of energetic resonance.

Reflexes could be described as nodes or control points on a particular current of energy. A correspondence is a harmonic that, when activated, may exert a controlling effect (if it is a reflex) but it may also modulate its related areas in a multitude of other ways. In a sense a reflex has a quite specific effect, whereas a harmonic correspondence is often more global and diverse in its effect.

Classification

There is a broad classification of correspondences as being either *involutionary* or *evolutionary* in nature. What this classification denotes is the process by which all the various correspondences are created.

An involutionary correspondence is created during the process of creation and incarnation into the world. It is symbolised by a downward pointing triangle. We can speak of a human being as having a soul that becomes involved into the world of matter when it takes on a physical form or body. The life energy, manifesting as the unfolding human consciousness, is involved in the world, in life and all its drama in such areas as; family, relationships, sexuality, work, and the health of the body.

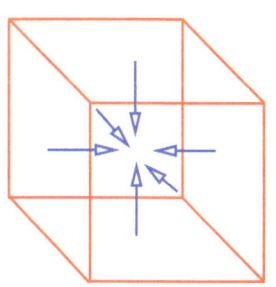

The involutionary focus of attention is inward on the self, where everything that happens in life is all about 'me'. It has a strong resonance with the foetal position in the womb. It is a position of protection such as when we present the strong, outer shell (back) of the body to the world. It can be thought of as a box in which all the sides are inward facing.

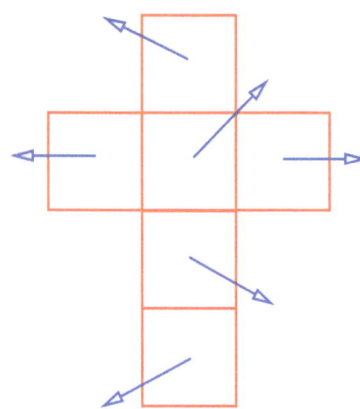

An evolutionary correspondence is created during the journey through life and the natural process of growth. A human being, composed of soul, consciousness and body, focusses attention back to its Source in spirit. This is symbolised by an upward pointing triangle. The evolutionary focus of attention is upward and outward away from the self, initially into the world and then finally back to a spiritual source. It has a strong resonance with the physical position of surrender when the arms are outstretched and the body arches backward into a cross shape. In this case, the box is opened out into a cross where the focus is outward.

Simple classifications of things in the world, such as animals into a specific genus and plants into specific phyla are common. In the same way, objects can be classified as either solids, liquids or gasses. This common process could simply be called labelling and most of the time we just take the names of things for granted without giving them much thought and the labels do not necessarily add to our understanding. However, the labelling of correspondences as either involutionary or evolutionary does have a specific relevance and application.

The average client is most often caught up in concerns about their health, life and relationships etc. For these patients, working with *involutionary correspondences* is going to be the most effective approach as these correspondences are most resonant with the focus of their attention. However, some patients will be on an evolutionary journey and the focus of their attention may, in large part, be far removed from the concerns of the world. Such a focus does not preclude the body from succumbing to physical challenges and accidents, but if you have such a client, then the use of *evolutionary correspondences* is going to be more effective in getting a resolution.

Sometimes, it is hard to know when a client has such an evolutionary focus to their attention as some will hide it. In the later part of life, after the mid sixties, there is actually an inherent shift in consciousness from involution to evolution. It is important to be aware of this because, even though an elder client may appear on the surface to still be caught up in the drama of life, underneath in the hidden recesses of their heart and soul, a very different focus of consciousness may be fully active.

Reflex Disturbance

What does the pain and discomfort at any reflex area be it on the foot, hand or indeed anywhere else in the body actually signify? The simple answer is that it indicates a disturbance of energy flow and activity in those sore or painful areas.

What this information does not delineate is whether or not the problem is a current issue in an active phase, a disturbance that is in the process of resolving itself or the very beginning of some new process within the energy body. In other words what is not indicated is the time factor involved. Is it a past issue heading for resolution, a current problem or the early showing of a future disturbance?

Chronic and Acute Conditions

If the reflexes in the upper body areas above the diaphragm are more tender than the corresponding reflexes beneath the diaphragm you are dealing with an acute condition or an acute phase of a chronic condition. If the reflexes below the diaphragm are more tender or sensitive than those above it then you have a chronic condition.

If you are working on an acute condition, it is most effective to work on the reflex correspondences above the diaphragm first, and moving down through all the various corresponding areas to those in the lower body. If you are dealing with a chronic condition, you work from the lower body reflexes upward finishing with the reflex correspondences in the head.

Precision versus Holonomic

There is a certain precision in aspects of the human body, particularly in a physical sense, when looking at the location of nerve pathways. There is also precision in terms of the location of the energetic pathways of the Chinese acupuncture meridians. When the whole body is condensed or telescoped down and reflected in the feet it is obvious that large organs such as the liver have quite a large area on the foot but most parts of the body have very small areas of correspondence in the feet. Over the years this has given rise to a precision approach to reflexology - the idea that you need to pinpoint the exact location of an organ as represented in the feet to give an effective treatment. The reflexology charts in most modern textbooks give very exact mapping of the related reflex areas on the hands and feet. That said, there are a great many variations within the foot reflexology charts that map the body onto the feet. Some are so different that it rather defies the imagination to believe that they are all accurate and correct. Yet practitioners who follow widely differing mappings get consistent effective results using the maps that they trained with. This is most probably due to the influence of the consciousness and intent of the practitioner upon the behaviour of the life energy within the therapist-client holonomic system rather than any inherent accuracy in the reflex maps they are using.

The life force worked with in the Holonomic approach is not limited to those frequencies of energy used in Chinese medicine that do follow precise pathways. The Holonomic perception is that life energy flows in very broad flow patterns, very similar, in fact, to the behaviour of water, which apart from flowing in relatively straight currents when bound by a channel, also flows in three dimensional spirals and eddies.

From a holonomic perspective, exact mappings and treatment strategies based upon a precision model are going are going to have their limitations as the area that needs unlocking maybe be half an inch or a centimetre above or below or to the left or right of where a precision mapping suggests the location of the reflex to work might be. This is because a piece of a large hologram, whilst containing all the information of the whole, is fuzzy, its resolution being lower. This is somewhat counter intuitive to the common experience of using some form of magnifying glass to enhance the visual sense as this seems to increase the detail and precision of the visual experience.

This fuzziness is actually one of the great challenges of the Holonomic approach. There is a certain intellectual insecurity inherent in it. A Holonomic treatment is a continuous exploration of multiple possibilities, where the therapist is ultimately guided by energetic response rather than by any intellectual understanding

The Web of Consciousness – Hidden Dynamics

It is easy to get bogged down in the minutiae of exactly where to put one's hands. In precision reflexology, the exact spot on which to work is of paramount importance, especially if you are working with a model that relates to nervous system correspondences. However, such narrowing of focus can mean losing, or in some cases never even seeing, the bigger picture that is so important in the Holonomic approach.

When we narrow our focus, we are in danger of obscuring all other perspectives. Each of us is part of a great picture and like every picture it has a background and a foreground as well as a focal point of attention. It is these perspectives that give the picture interest, depth and complexity, which in turn affords us more information and understanding.

In Holonomic Reflexology, we understand that even though our attention may be drawn to one specific area of the body, due to the fact that we are interacting with the person's energy, there will be ramifications and reverberations throughout their entire field. In other words, the effect is not confined to any single organ, nerve pathway or zone.

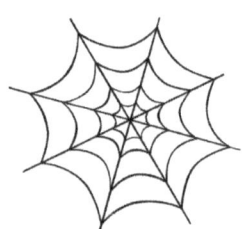

Think, for a moment, of a spider web. This intricate structure, passively hanging on fine, gossamer threads, immediately transmits any vibration from say, a wayward insect, throughout the entire web alerting the builder lying in wait under the shade of a leaf. This analogy is a good approximation of what happens in our living energy field of consciousness when one part of our body/mind becomes stimulated or impinged upon by either internal or external forces. The vibrations created are immediately transmitted throughout the field of consciousness and the consequences of that initial onslaught registered everywhere at once.

In practice, this can mean that, problems cannot be solved in isolation, we must recognise that in order to resolve them we have to view them as systemic. That is to say, all problems are both interconnected and interdependent. To solve any persistent problem requires a shift in perspective, a more holistic view.

To be effective as a therapist one needs to be something of a detective. Like a detective, you need to get the whole story by questioning everybody, you look for clues, you try to discover hidden motives and establish a time-line, until eventually you expose the culprit.

The person who sits before us in our therapy room or graciously lies upon our treatment couch is not a condition, (today I have 2 bad backs and a stomach ulcer to see). They do not exist in isolation, although that may seem to be the case for the short time that they spend with us. They have family, friends, acquaintances, all of whom they are constantly interacting with and being influenced by.

When we complain of a headache it is easy to focus on the problem as being just in the head. We may put away the book we are reading, massage our temples or take a pain killer, yet if we take a more holistic perspective, we may begin to understand that our headache has more to do with our inability to digest the heavy meal we have just eaten; or the muscle strain in our neck from hours of reading; or high blood pressure; or our unexpressed anger at our boss. To solve the problem of the headache, all these different perspectives need to be taken into account and resolved in order for us to become pain free.

We can expand this holistic viewpoint to encompass the recognition of the intrinsic value of all living beings and that the human race is but one strand of a great web of life. That is to say, as living beings we consist of a living system of networks that is constantly interacting with other network systems. We do not exist in isolation. We are a part of much greater networks.

Beyond our own energy field, there is the field of our personal environment – our family, friends, the whole of humanity. As a person makes shifts and changes, so too, do all these other people to whom they are energetically connected. That same person is also a part of a bigger network, that of society and of the web of humanity.

Even beyond the backdrop of humanity, there is the greater network of Nature. It is so easy to forget that we are an integral part of the natural world. Beyond this still, is the even greater energy field of the conscious universe that we exist within and which constantly interpenetrates our own. Conscious networks within conscious networks, all interconnected and interdependent.

Setting the Scene

Before any important undertaking, it is essential to adequately prepare and this also applies to beginning a Holonomic Reflexology session. You can think of it as preparing the scene before a performance or an artist contemplating a blank canvas before beginning to paint.

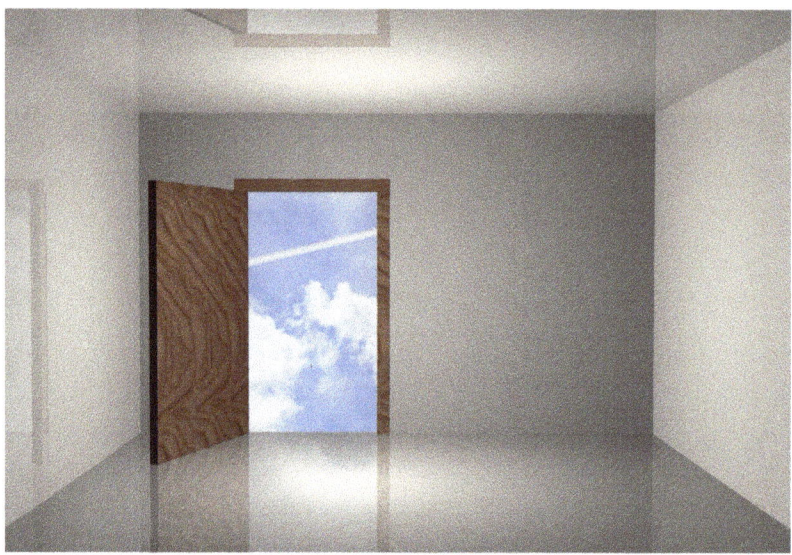

The space in which you are working is a stage for you and your client. Both of you will be present in a 'bubble' of energy in which all interaction and communication takes place. Your presence, calm openness and relaxed attention will encourage the unfolding of the healing that will occur.

If you are a reflexologist, you could begin with a relaxed palm contact on top on the client's feet or cupping their heels. If you are a massage therapist or other type of bodyworker and use a bodywork table, you could cradle the client's head or hold their shoulders. As you hold the client's body you begin to open an awareness of your own life energy. You can start with the physical sense of your own body by allowing yourself to become aware of the pressure on your pelvis as you sit, or on your feet, if you are standing. Then include the feeling of your clothing against your skin and allow yourself to become aware of what you see and hear around you. Notice if you are using broad or narrow focus and if you are internally or externally orientated or if you are shifting from one to another. From these deepening physical cues you will find yourself easily shifting to an awareness of the energy movement within your body and any streaming or pulsatory activity therein. You should always allow for the possibility that, at an energetic level, there may be a profound stillness inside you.

Then open up an awareness of the energy you sense within your client's body. Allow yourself to be aware of your own internal energetic activity and the client's own energetic process simultaneously, as you consciously acknowledge that you and the client form a conjoint entity. Once you have done this, open up your awareness to include the physical space that you are working within, becoming aware of both you and the client as being within a larger space. Sometimes it is useful to shift your awareness momentarily to all the corners (or walls, including the floor and ceiling) of the room.

At this stage you can let this awareness process move into the background of your consciousness, as you begin to focus on the foreground of the actual work you need to do on the client's body. Just because you shift your awareness to the foreground activity it does not follow that all the preparatory scene setting disappears or is lost. Just as in a stage play, the backdrop once placed, persists throughout the performance until it is changed.

This whole awareness process is the creation of a framework within which all the therapeutic activity takes place and is bound by. If you are a reflexologist or aromatherapist who uses reflexology as a diagnostic tool, beginning any session with this scene setting process will take your work to an entirely different level.

Holonomic Treatment

A Holonomic treatment of any body part or organ occurs in two phases. The first is an assessment procedure to ascertain which particular correspondences will be most effective in achieving a resolution. The second is the creation of energetic coherence between the areas.

Assessment

One hand is placed lightly over the body part or organ needing attention and the other hand on one of the many other corresponding areas. The hand on the problem area is the *listening hand*. After taking a moment or two to establish a baseline of physical and energetic sensation experienced under the listening hand, the other *activating hand* is placed, in turn, on any of the corresponding reflex areas. At every connection, wait for a reaction under the listening hand. By keeping a hand on the problem area and touching all the areas that reflex to it, the effect of each reflex can be monitored. Most commonly, there will be one specific reflex correspondence that 'unlocks' the problem area. When the correct reflex is found, the right key as it were, a strong reaction under the listening hand is usually experienced. Any significant change of sensation is important and is indicative that a dynamic connection exists between these two areas. A systematic approach to checking the corresponding reflexes is advised, possibly starting from the feet upward although you can create your own sequence. Remember to think 3-dimensionally (top/bottom, front/back, left/right) when checking all the correspondences.

You may find that more than one corresponding area will give a response under the listening hand. In general, you would focus your subsequent treatment upon the correspondence that gives the greatest response.

In some cases, you may find a strong area of correspondence in the first two or three areas contacted. Then the question arises as to whether you should continue checking all the other corresponding areas. This is a personal choice, you can check the other areas but usually, it is enough to work with the first dynamic connection you experience.

Creating Coherence

To create coherence between the body part or organ and a dynamic correspondence, an alternating activation of the two areas is used. The actual body contacts can be made with the palms or fingers. It involves stimulating one contact area for about 15 - 20 seconds and then simply holding that contact as you stimulate the other area for approximately the same amount of time. Alternate the stimulation back and forth between the two contacts for 2-3 minutes. Finally, both contacts are held for 1-2 minutes whilst listening for the energetic response. This technique 'pulses' the energy back and forth between the two areas, which aids in the establishment of a coherent energy flow.

If the problem area presented with a degree of pain, you can palpate to check if there is a reduction in sensitivity. If there is no change in the level of pain you may need to check for and treat any other dynamic connections. For other types of conditions when functional improvement can only be assessed through client feedback, the process may need to continue over a number of full sessions.

Due to the existence of hidden dynamics many therapists will prefer not to focus their attention upon just the presenting symptoms. However, from a practical perspective in, for example, cases of injury, this is completely valid as a treatment strategy. It is also a useful approach when a problem is in its early stages and any deeper forces have yet to come into play.

Hidden Dynamics

As so many of the problems that a client brings to the treatment room have hidden dynamics, it is important to address these in a practical way. This can be done by eliciting specific information from the client and helping them to acknowledge that there may be other factors playing a part in their problems. Having acknowledged the possibility of such influences, it may then be possible to help them to see their problem in a different light and open up the possibility of a new kind of transformative action within their life.

However, such an approach may fall outside the scope of a therapist's training and experience. Even if a therapist has the required level of communication skills, a client can be unwilling to accept the possibility of such hidden influences, though it can be obvious to the therapist that there are both internal and/or external factors at play. In either of these two situations it is possible to influence these dynamics through *intent*.

In every day life, intent, though common, is often momentary and frequently fails. We intend to do something, only to lack the will to follow through. The world, it is said, is full of good intentions, yet few come to fruition. The intent utilised in Holonomic Reflexology is specific. It is a relaxed mental focus on the *resolution of all hidden dynamics* which is initially held in the foreground of the therapist's thoughts at the beginning of the session. As the session continues, this intent is naturally displaced by other thoughts relating to treatment strategy etc., so it is important that it is re-visited regularly throughout the session, for a few moments at a time, to ensure that it stays active and energised.

The web of consciousness that every human being exists within is essentially an energy based phenomenon. The individual threads of the web are energetic tendrils that exchange information at an unconscious level creating complex feedback loops that can alter thoughts and modify behaviour. Both therapist and the client have their own webs of consciousness but when they come together a new and much larger field of consciousness that behaves as a complex adaptive system is created. One of the functions of the therapist's clear intent is that it acts as a filter that prevents a flow of influence from the client to the therapist, meaning that the practitioner just acts as a catalyst inputting new information but does not become directly involved in any new feedback loops that the treatment creates.

Simultaneously holding the clear intent, as well as an awareness of the three dimensional web of connections that the client exists within, allows the energetic shifts to ramify throughout the client's web.

The web of interaction that is the client's world is composed of many smaller systems nested within each other that create the total adaptive system that is their life. A change in the behaviour of even one small part of one nested system can, through iteration, affect the behaviour of the whole in a dramatic way. So, as the therapist affects the inter relationship of the life energy as it plays through the client's emotions, thoughts and physical body, the influence will ripple outward through the energetic threads to all the other areas of client's life in exactly the same way as a small pebble dropped into a still pond sends ripples throughout the whole pond.

Alternate Treatment Strategy

Outside of a specifically Holonomic treatment approach as outlined earlier, there are a number of other ways of working. These approaches may be more familiar to reflexologists. The strategies listed below are not the only possibilities.

1. Work 3-dimensionally. For example, when working the gall bladder reflexes on the feet, simultaneous contacts would be made on both feet. The gall bladder reflex on the right foot is stimulated whilst stimulating the mirrored correspondence on the left foot (left/right) at the same time.

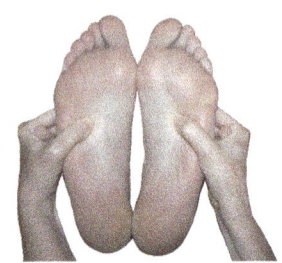

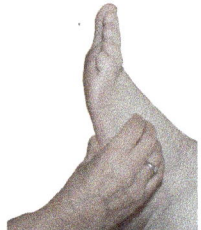

Using a light grip between thumb and forefinger of each hand, contact the gall bladder reflex on the soles of the feet with the thumbs, which represents the front of the body (front/back) and the mirror reflex on the top of each foot with the forefinger. (The sole of foot and top of foot represent the front and back of the body respectively.)

Finally, to affect a top/bottom contact, contact is made between the gall bladder reflex on the right foot with any corresponding area above the diaphragm line on the foot. The same is done on the mirror reflexes on the left foot(top/bottom). The top/bottom connection could also be made diagonally from the reflex on one foot to the corresponding area on the top of the other foot.

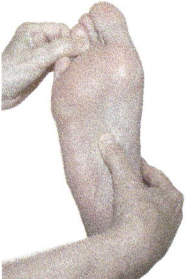

2. Connect the painful areas on the feet to the relevant body part or organ. This would normally be done using an alternating activation of the two areas in question. For example, a painful kidney reflex on the right foot would be held with a finger or thumb whilst the other hand is placed over the anatomical location of the right kidney. Then alternately stimulate of the foot reflex and kidney for approximately for 2-3 minutes. Then wait for a shift in the energy before checking for a reduction in sensitivity.

3. Connect the disturbed reflex areas on the feet to all their other related reflex areas and correspondences. Assess the degree of pain or discomfort at each reflex or correspondence, giving particular time and attention to those areas which are most painful. Use alternating contacts. In this strategy the organ or body part that shows up as disturbed in the assessment of the foot reflexes is not addressed directly but is only worked *indirectly* through all its corresponding reflex areas.

The 3-dimensional approach should also be used in strategies 2 and 3. For example, when connecting the gall bladder reflex on the right foot to the gall bladder, a connection should also be made from the foot reflex to the mirror correspondences of the gall bladder on the left side of the torso as well as on the back of the body.

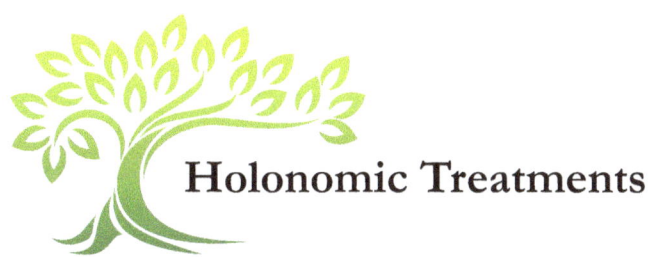

Holonomic Treatments

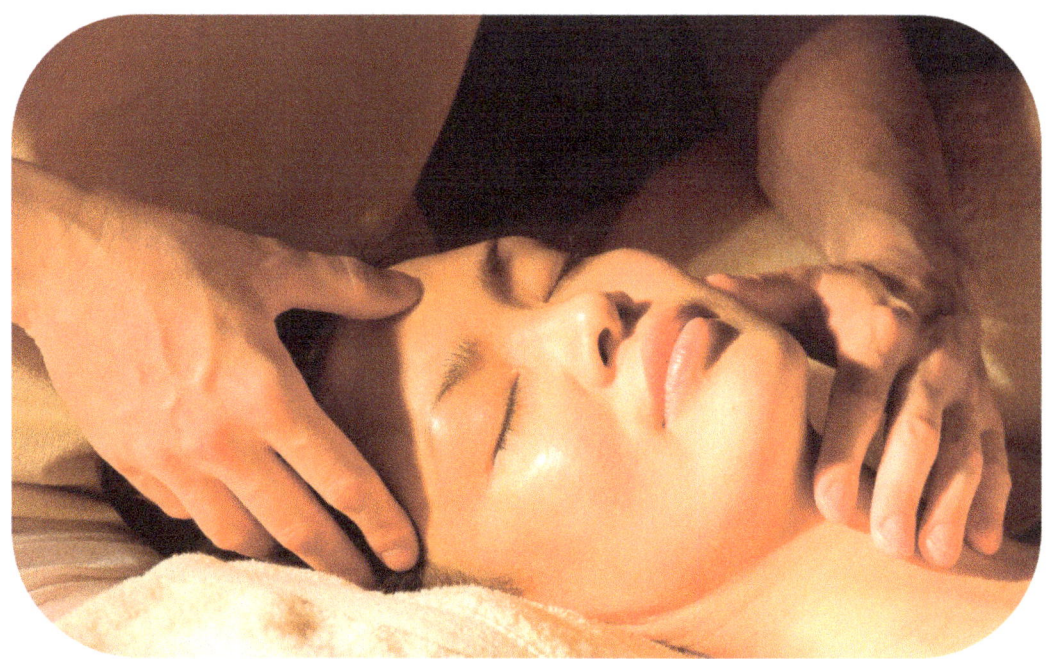

Holonomic Treatment

Constitutional Treatment

Holonomic Foot Reflexology Session

Diaphragm Treatment

Organ Treatments

Spinal Correspondences

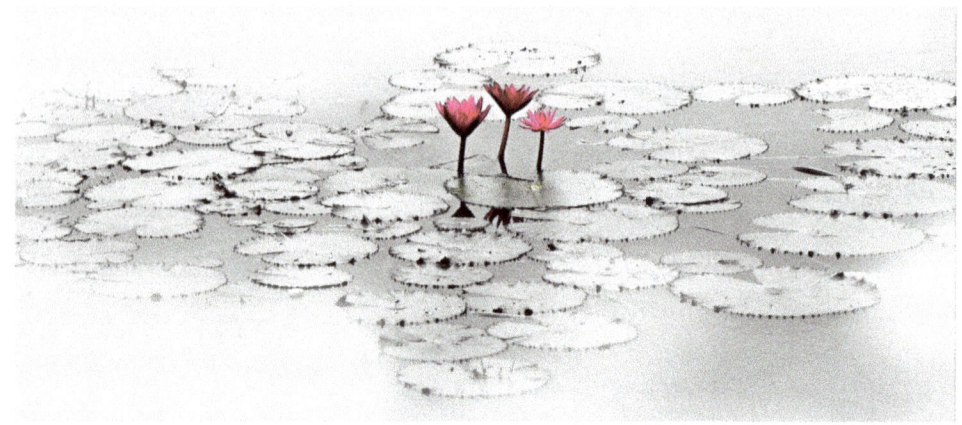

The treatments that follow are suggested ways of working. They include some of the reflexes and correspondences mapped in Holonomic Reflexology but not all. Study of the charts in the section on Cartography and the organ charts that follow will enable the practitioner to recognise the many reflexes and correspondences available to them and assesment, as well experience, will tell which ones are the most effective in any given circumstance.

> "Your heart is full of fertile seeds, waiting to sprout. Just as a lotus flower springs from the mire to bloom splendidly, the interaction of the cosmic breath causes the flower of the spirit to bloom and bear fruit in this world."
>
> Morihei Ueshiba

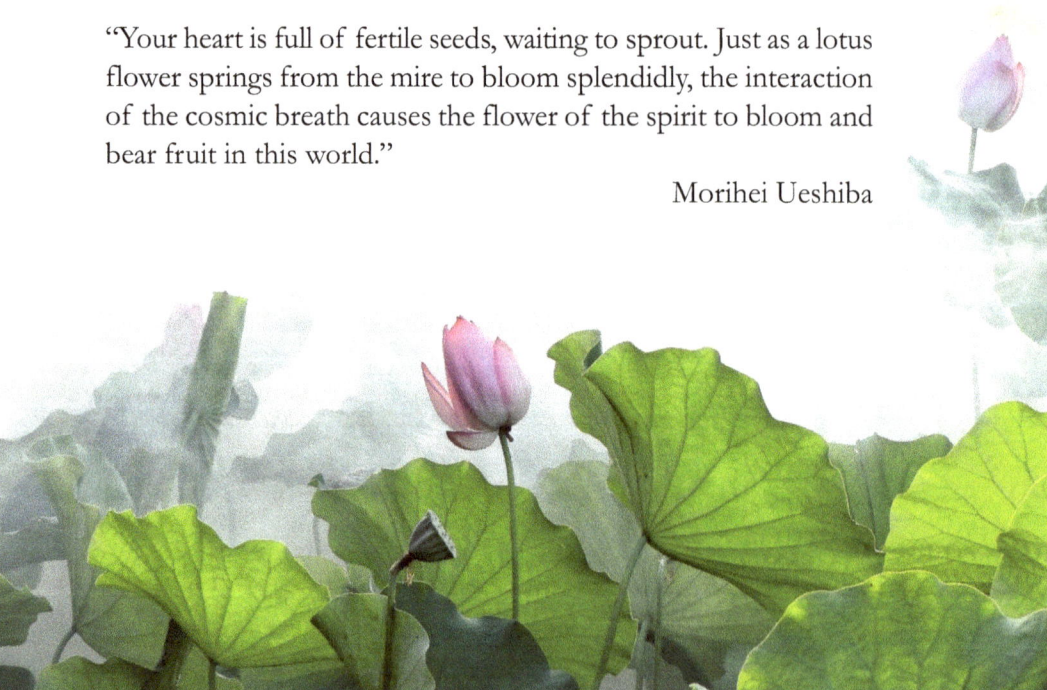

Holonomic Treatment

The following sequence is the basic *framework* for any Holonomic Reflexology treatment. This framework is not a declaration of exactly how things should be done, as any experienced therapist will, over time, modify the work to match their understanding. However, this particular framework is an excellent place to begin.

Preparation

These holds allow you to tune into the client, set the scene and engage your holonomic perception.

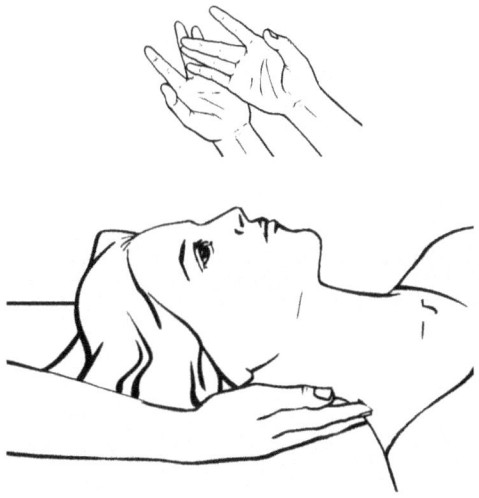

Hold the hands as illustrated. Then slide them under the head so that the palms of the hands cradle the occiput. The index fingers should connect to the side of the neck. Soften the hands to establish a good connection with the head and remain relaxed whilst tuning into the sensations of the client's energy. Hold this position until you sense the person relax. Watch for physical signs such as a deepening of the breath and a softening of facial expression.

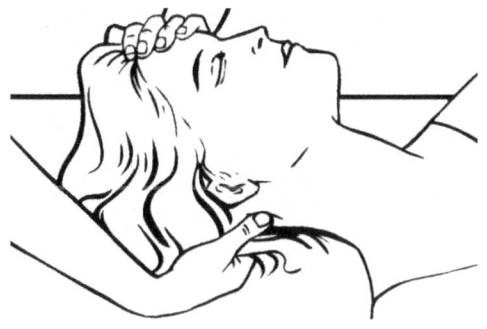

Now slide the right hand under the occiput and gently mould the left hand to the forehead with the left thumb in the area of the anterior fontanel on the top of the head. Keep the contact light. This hold harmonises the relationship between the front and back of the body.

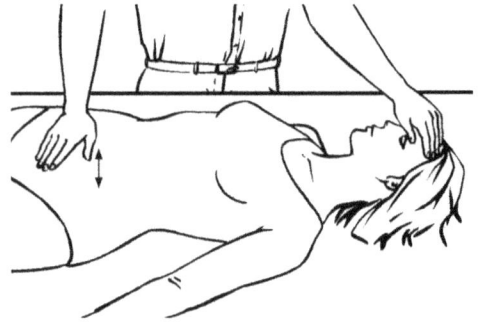

Next place your left hand lightly on the forehead and your right hand on the lower abdomen, between the iliac crests of the pelvis. Begin to rock the pelvis. Your hand should remain relaxed as you make a slight push across the pelvis, provided your hand is relaxed you should feel the pelvis recoil back toward you and then you can push gently again. Repeat until a rhythm is established. Move too fast and you will end up jiggling, press too firmly in to the body and you will end up punching into the pelvis. The rocking is continuous and once a rhythm has been established, just like pushing a swing, very little effort is required to keep the pelvis in motion. Rock for at least a minute and then stop and hold the hands still until you sense a coherent energy flow between them.

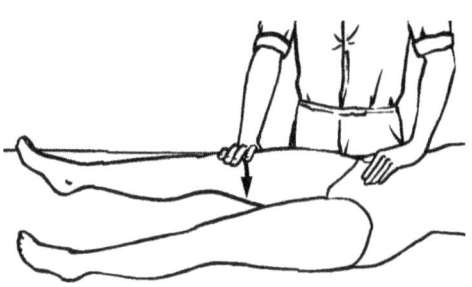

Now move your hands down the body and place the upper hand so that it cups the iliac crest of the pelvis whilst the lower hand rests on the outside of the leg just above the knee. Keeping the upper hand still, roll the leg inward with the lower hand. Do not push and pull. Simply roll the leg inward and let the recoil return it to its normal position before rolling again. Once a steady rhythm has been established, continue to rock the leg for about 30 seconds and then stop. Hold the hands still to establish a coherent flow.

Repeat on the other leg. Then stroke down both legs several times keeping the hands relaxed with fingers spread a little as you draw down the five energetic zones of the legs.

Specifics

At this stage you would work on any specific reflexes or correspondences, as required, to address the client's needs.

Closing

Holonomic treatment always finishes by creating a balance of the right and left sides of the energy body of the head

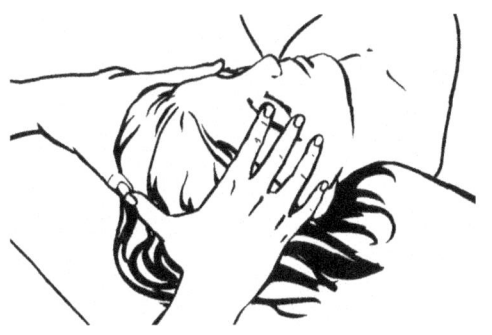

Gently place thumbs on the anterior fontanel on the top of the head and place the fingers equidistant on either side of the head. The contact should be light. Wait for energetic coherence.

The Constitution

A person's constitution is their innate or inherent strength and vitality. A strong constitution enables a person to recover easily from illness. Constitution varies from person to person and is dependent on a number of both passive, congenital (genetic) factors and active environmental influences. Nutrition, metabolism, organ function, emotionality are just a few of the things that determine and influence how susceptible we may be to pathogenic factors. In times of prolonged stress our constitution can weaken, or through no fault of our own, we simply have a less than robust constitution. Either way, a boost to our ability to deal with illness and stress by strengthening our constitution is not only helpful but a necessary part of any treatment regimen.

Constitutional treatment is a fundamental part of Holonomic Reflexology. The constitution is always supported first before commencing any other treatment. Astrology has a vital part to play with regard to a person's constitution as the element that relates to their sun sign is the most active factor in determining the energetic quality of their constitution.

To be able to activate the constitution it is necessary to know the client's sign of the Zodiac or sun sign (commonly misnamed their star sign). Armed with this piece of information, we can then link the sign to its element (see p. 79) and then to its related elemental centre (see p. 97). For example, if the sun sign is in Aries which is a Fire sign, the elemental centre is the solar plexus. The related fire signs of Leo and Sagittarius complete this particular astrological triad. Each astrological triad has three related body parts in this case they are eyes, solar plexus and thighs. All this information is used in a constitutional treatment.

Constitutional Treatment

This sequence is a specific for stimulating a person's underlying constitution. Before the bodywork, establish the person's sun sign, element, elemental centre (and location) as well as the related body parts.

The example that follows is for a client born under the sign of Gemini, Libra or Aquarius. These signs are related to the air element meaning that the air centre in the chest needs to be activated. This is performed in three phases, firstly, the stimulation of the second toes and the index fingers. This is done by gently squeezing and pulling on the fingers and toes in a rhythmic 'milking' manner. Secondly, connecting the fingers and toes to the air element centre in the chest. Thirdly, connect shoulders, kidneys and ankles which are the body parts that relate to the air element

When working with the other astrological signs and their related element simply work the related finger and toe to its elemental centre according to the chart opposite.

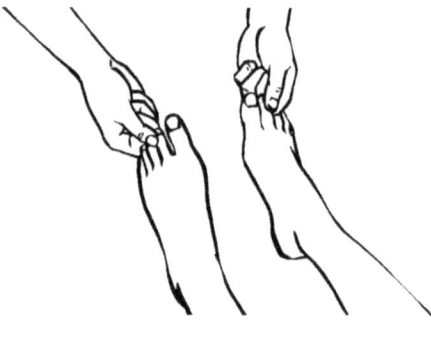

Begin to stimulate the air element by working the top and bottom of both second toes simultaneously with the milking action. After 2-3 minutes stop and hold the toes feeling for coherence.

If there is little or no response continue the stimulation of the toes. This may take several minutes as they can be congested.

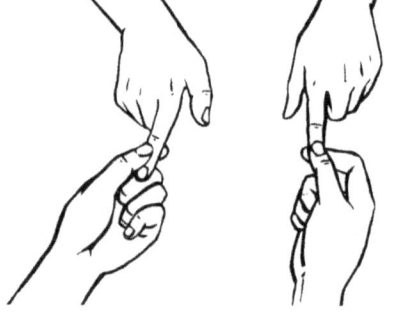

Now take hold of both forefingers and perform the same action that was carried out on the toes. After 1-2 minutes stop and wait for an energetic response.

Finger and Toe Relationships to the Elemental Centres

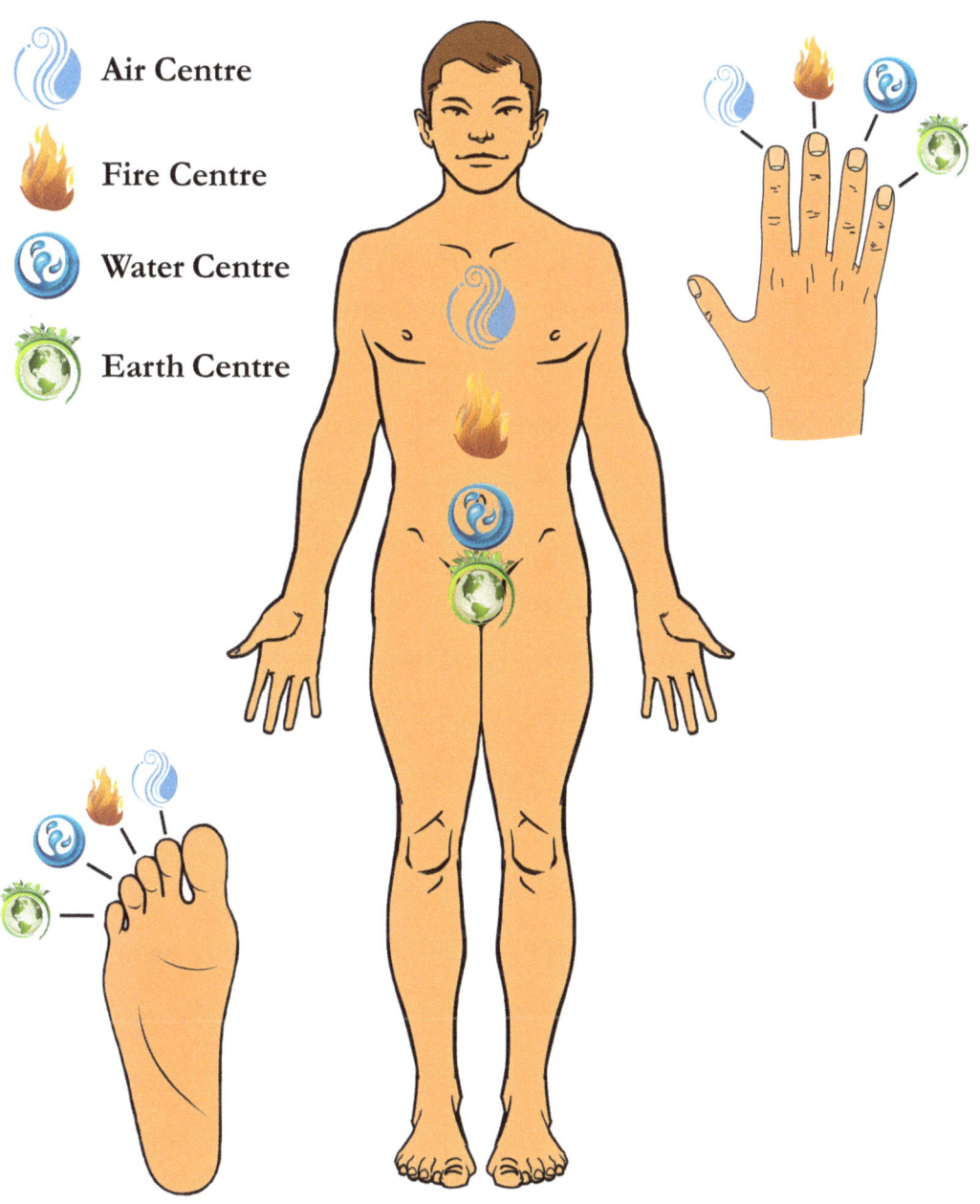

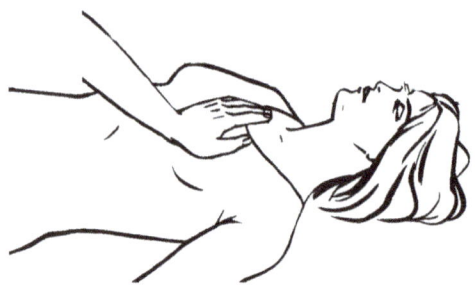

Then, holding the second toe, place the other hand on the air element centre in the middle of the chest. Stimulate the toe as before, alternating with a gentle rocking of the chest toward the head with the other hand for 1-2 minutes. Stop and leave the hands in place sensing any changes. Then, leaving the hand on the air element centre, take hold of the forefinger and stimulate as described above. This procedure is then repeated on the other side of the body. Watch for any physical shifts such as changes in breathing, body movements and attend to any global energy responses. (see p. 32).

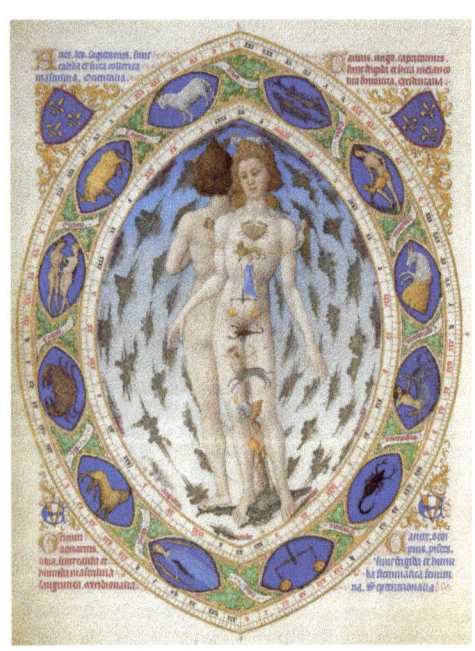

Now connect the body parts associated with the astrological triad of the air element as shown on the chart on the opposite page.

Stand to the side of the body and mould one hand to the ankle (Aquarius/air element). Slide the other hand under the body in the area of the kidney (Libra/air element) on the same side. Hold both contacts. Then move both hands, placing one hand on the shoulder (Gemini/air element) and again sliding the other hand under the body to the kidney area moulding both contacts to body. Finally, leaving the hand on the shoulder, take the other hand and mould it to the ankle on the same side again. Repeat the sequence on the other side of the body.

All of the contacts are held for about 1 minute as you sense for energetic coherence.

Finish with the closing head hold.

Elemental Body Correspondences

"The art of the true healer must be to balance man with Nature, tune him into the greater energy field, so all the elements can flow and function. That is how Nature heals".
Polarity Therapy - Dr. Randolph Stone - Vol II, Book 5, p. 61

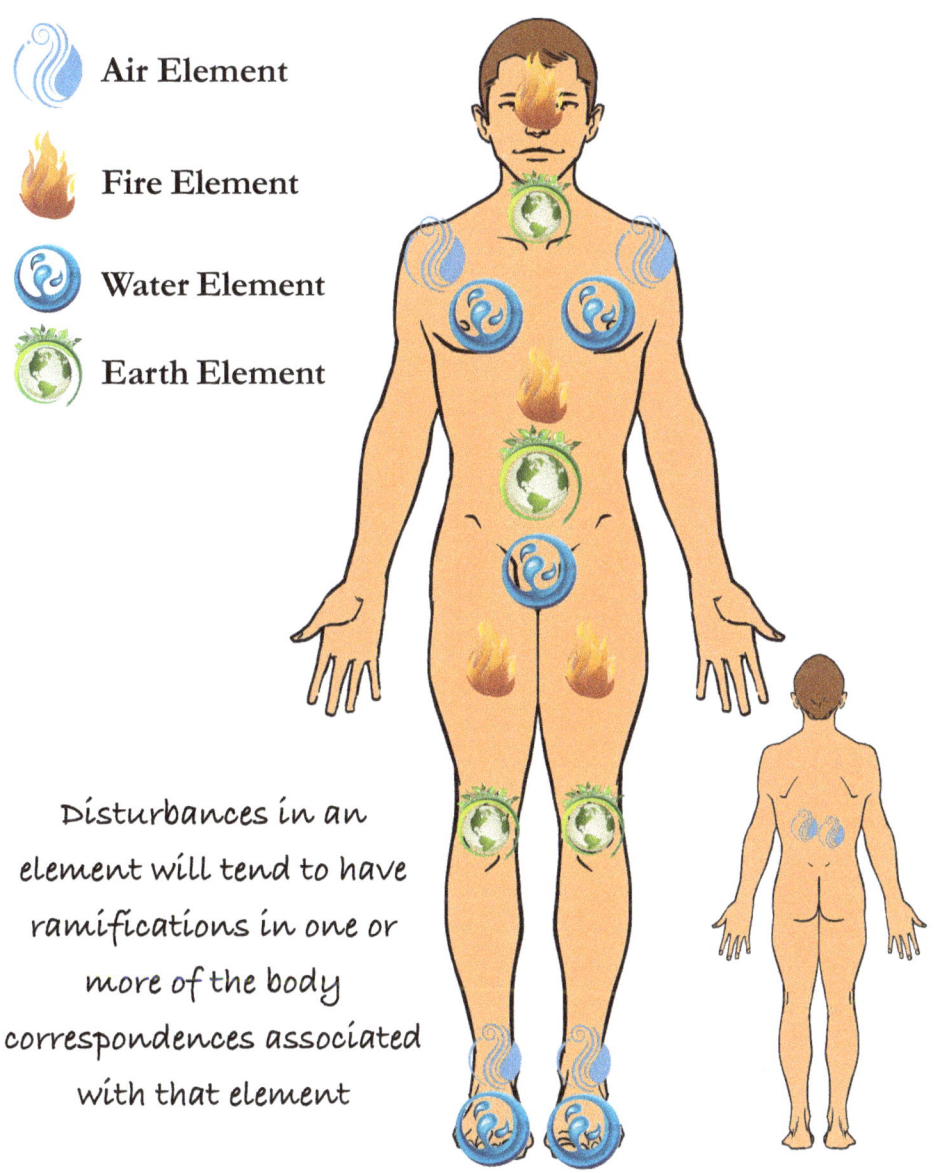

- Air Element
- Fire Element
- Water Element
- Earth Element

Disturbances in an element will tend to have ramifications in one or more of the body correspondences associated with that element

See Astrological Sign, Element & Body Correspondences p. 79

Further Astrological Correspondences

There is also a relationship between the joints of the fingers and toes and the body parts related to the astrological signs of that element. Thus, the first joint of the forefingers and toes relate to Gemini (shoulders), the first joint of the middle fingers and toes to Aries (head/eyes), the first joint of the ring fingers and toes to Cancer (the breast area) and the first joint of the little fingers and toes to Taurus (the neck). In the same way, the middle joint of each finger and toe relates to the second astrological sign in the same element and the lower joint of the fingers and toes relates to the last of the signs in the same element. Any pain or discolouration in any of these areas can be an important indicator of energetic disturbance.

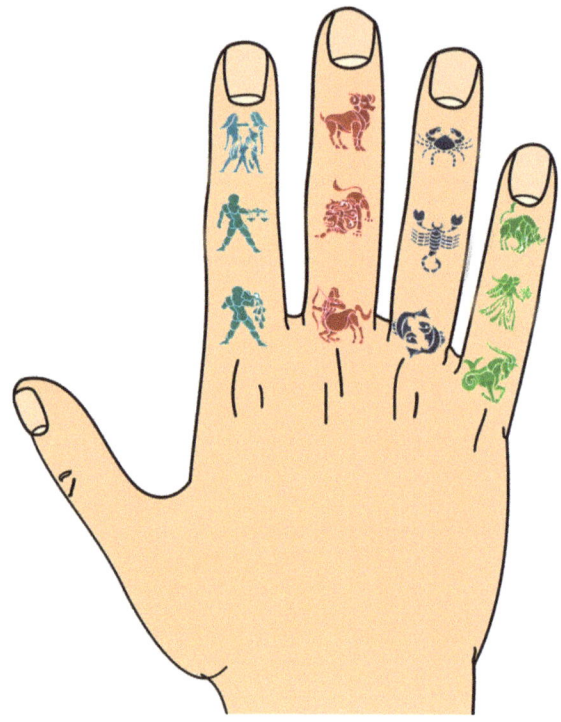

★ Beyond the context of constitutional treatment you may wish to work on the different elements and their astrological body correspondences when there is a disturbance in any of the body parts related to an element.

Holonomic Foot Reflexology Session

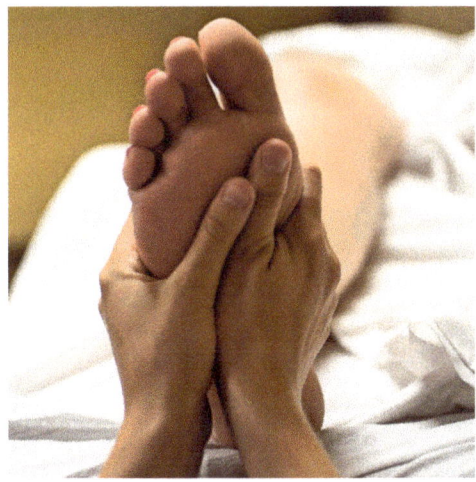

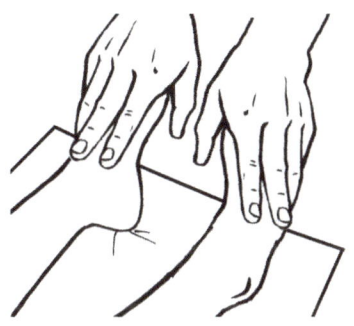

Begin by lightly holding both feet to activate the right/left geometric relationships and tune into the energy that you experience. You can rest your hands on top of the feet as illustrated opposite or as an alternative, you can cradle both heels. Use which ever contact feels most effective in terms of your holonomic perception.

Then, placing the hands gently on the knees, pull them slowly down the legs and off the ends of the toes to activate the reflex zones in the legs. Repeat 2 or 3 times.

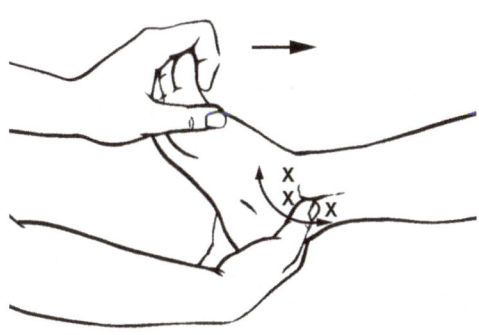

Now wrap your hand over the toes as illustrated. At the same time cradle the heel in the palm of your other hand. Then flex the foot by pushing the ball of the foot toward the head. Let the foot return to its natural position. Then press gently on one of areas shown with an x in the figure opposite. Alternate between these two movements in a rhythmic fashion, moving back and forth in an arc around the inside of the heel and continuing this stimulation for 2 minutes. Keep both hands in contact with the foot at all times.

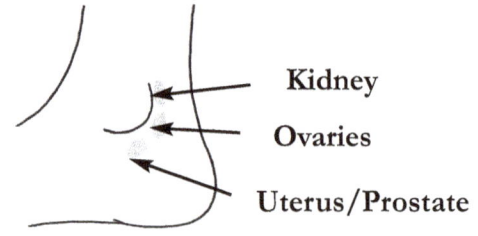

Kidney
Ovaries
Uterus/Prostate

This technique stimulates the pelvis in general. You may, of course, adopt the same technique to contact specific organ reflexes areas such as the ovaries or uterus. In this case instead of pressing around the lower arc of the ankle bone you would focus on just one area.

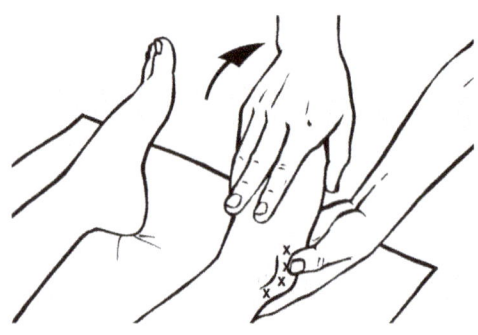

Next place your hand over the top of foot with your other hand once again cradling the heel, but this time with the thumb contacting the outside of the heel bone. Extend the ankle by gently pushing down on the foot. As the foot returns to its natural position press on the points around the outside of the heel in an arc. Continue with this rhythmic alternate stimulation working systematically back and forth around the heel for 2 minutes. Again keep both hands in contact with the foot at all times.

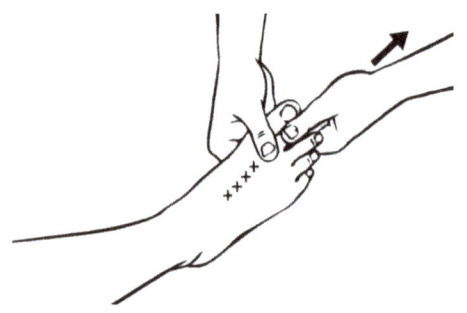

This next technique stretches the tendons of the feet which can often be contracted. Take the first toe between your thumb and first finger and stretch it toward you then relax the toe and squeeze the tendon top and bottom with the same fingers of your other hand.

Repeat this alternating stimulation in a rhythmic fashion working up along the length of the tendon 2 or 3 times. Repeat the procedure for each toe, including the big toe.

Now hold the foot and sense for energetic coherence.

Repeat on the other foot.

 By pressing the top and bottom of the foot simultaneously the front/back geometric relationship of the whole body is activated

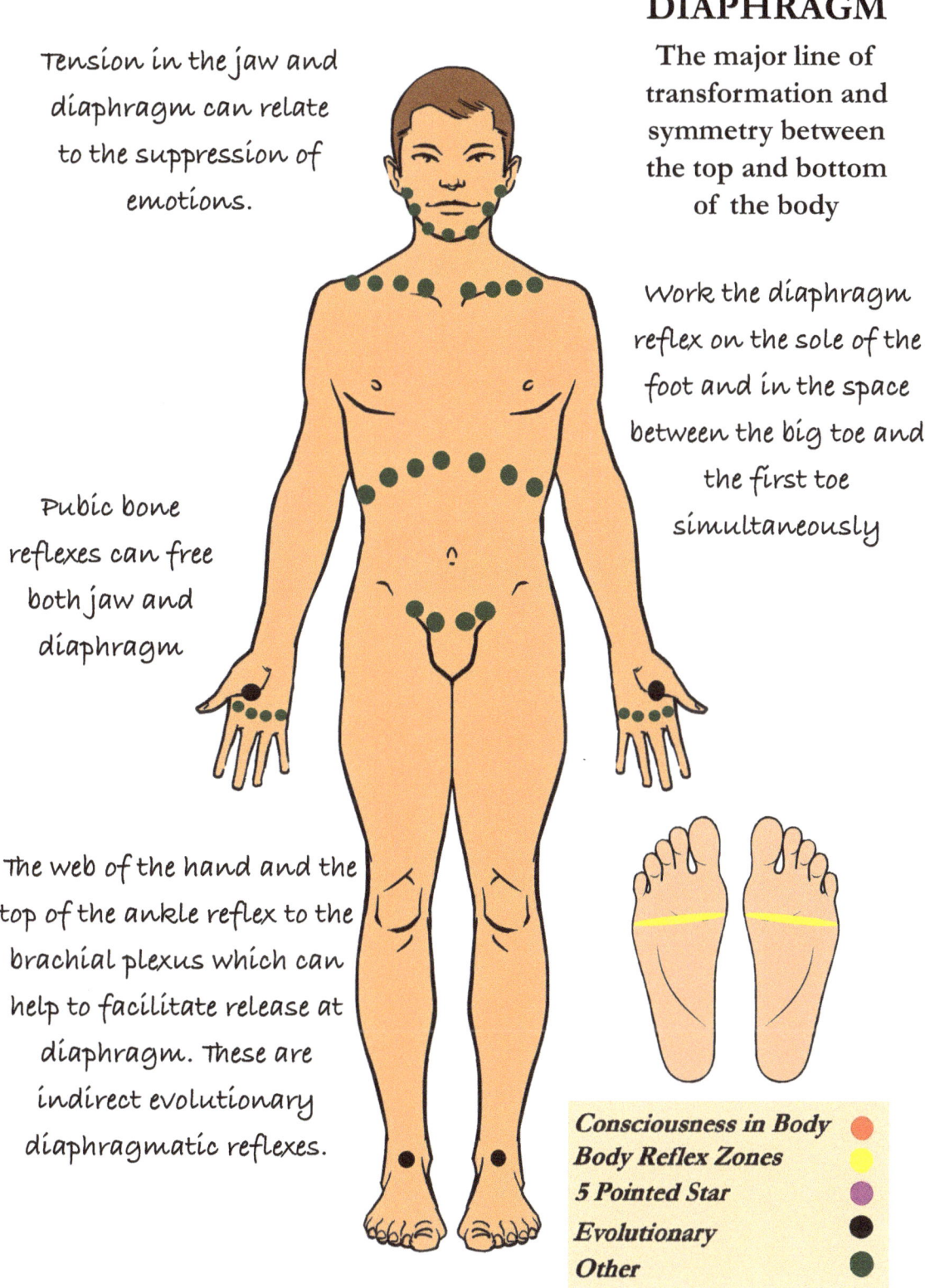

Diaphragm Treatment

The diaphragm is a double domed sheet of muscle that separates the thoracic cavity from the abdominal cavity. It is an important area of the body and is worthy of attention in a range of conditions. Obviously, it plays an important part in respiration, but it also serves to massage the digestive organs; aids in the lifting of the chest at each in breath which affects the functioning of the thyroid gland; aids in the return flow of blood and lymph from the lower body and, of course, brings fresh oxygen into the body to vitalise it.

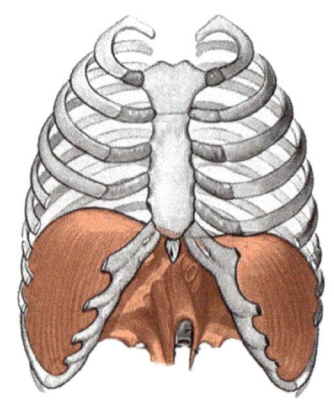

The diaphragm has an important, but not always helpful part to play in locking down strong emotions in the body and a tense diaphragm can affect the posture of the body and impede the functions of the heart and abdominal organs. Most people breathe poorly and this can lead to a lot of health problems.

The diaphragm forms the major transverse line of transformation in the body.

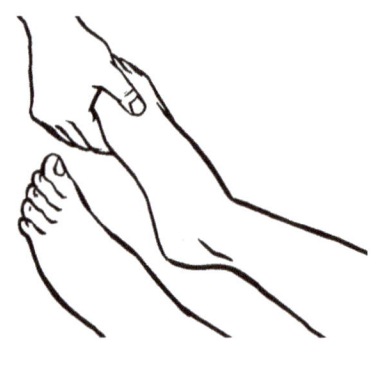

By working the area between the tendons of the big toe and the first toe we are stimulating the shoulder girdle which is a major correspondence to the diaphragm and will help to increase breathing capacity. Whilst the thumb works into this area, the forefinger works into the diaphragm reflex on the sole of the foot. Both feet need to be stimulated in this way. This can be done simultaneously by crossing the hands - left hand working the right foot and vice versa.

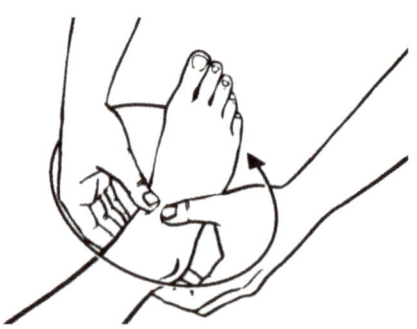

Then place both thumbs in the indentation on the top of the right ankle, which is another diaphragmatic correspondence. Circle both thumbs a few times clockwise and then counter clockwise and then hold for coherence. Repeat on the left ankle.

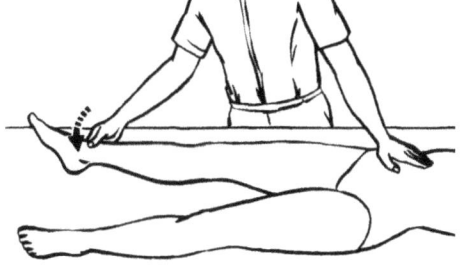

Placing one thumb on the indentation on top of the ankle, rock the leg inward several times alternating with working under the lower ribs with either finger tips or the side of the thumb. Begin working near the centre of the diaphragm on that side and gradually work outward until the area relaxes.

Keep your hand relaxed and direct the fingers or thumb upward under the ribs toward the diaphragm. It can be helpful to co-ordinate your directional impulses up under the ribs with the client's out breath. This is done on both sides of the body. Sense the energy at each area.

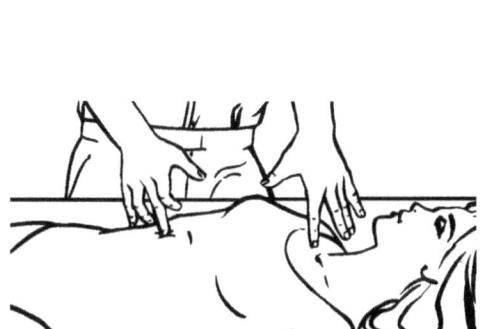

Then place the middle finger of the right hand near the centre of the body just below the ribcage on the diaphragm and the forefinger of the left hand on the corresponding diaphragmatic reflex point on the same energy current line just below the clavicle. Gently simulate both areas alternately, wait for energetic coherence, then move the fingers along the ribcage and the clavicle to the next zone or line of energy out toward the outside of the body. Treat all five lines of energy.

Repeat the same process on the other side of the body making contacts with the middle finger of the right hand at the clavicle and the forefinger of the left hand at the diaphragm.

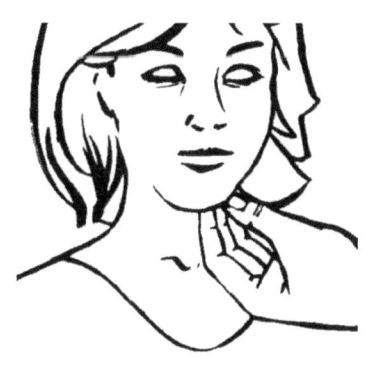

Lightly grip the jaw between finger and thumb and stimulate in a circular motion whilst alternating with a stimulation of the diaphragm with the fingers. Move the contacts from the centre outward along the lines of energy at both jaw and diaphragm, allowing the energy to respond at each area. Repeat on the other side of the body.

Organ Treatments

What follows are charts of correspondences and suggestions for working some of the major organs of the body. There many more correspondences and reflexes to the organs than are shown on the charts. The specific correspondences illustrated are to simply stimulate your creativity and imagination. The correspondences shown are mostly drawn from the five pointed star, the body zones (vertical and horizontal) and the consciousness in the body chart. These charts are the most useful ones to refer to when treating any problem. They can be augmented by working further correspondences.

It is important to note that the charts do not show all the possible *mirror reflexes* which are an important aspect of the powerful left-right symmetry in the human body. Taking the gall bladder as an example, it has exact mirrored reflexes on the left side of the torso over the stomach. It is possible for a strong gall bladder disturbance to cause issues with the stomach function which will show up as sensitivity in the stomach reflexes. In this case, the cause of the sensitivity of the stomach reflexes is actually the gall bladder..

Your knowledge of locational anatomy and organ size is vital to Holonomic Reflexology. It would be ineffective to connect a gall bladder reflex to the middle of the abdomen, the listening hand needs to be over the actual gall bladder. The various techniques illustrated are, in no way, a statement of exactly how you should work with these organs and their correspondences.

The only way to master Holonomic Reflexology is to immerse yourself in the charts, to really study them and then experiment with all the different correspondences.

Why should we be concerned with symmetry? In the first place, symmetry is fascinating to the human mind, and everyone likes objects or patterns that are in some way symmetrical. It is an interesting fact that nature often exhibits certain kinds of symmetry in the objects we find in the world around us. Perhaps the most symmetrical object imaginable is a sphere, and nature is full of spheres—stars, planets, water droplets in clouds. The crystals found in rocks exhibit many different kinds of symmetry, the study of which tells us some important things about the structure of solids. Even the animal and vegetable worlds show some degree of symmetry, although the symmetry of a flower or of a bee is not as perfect or as fundamental as is that of a crystal.

But our main concern here is not with the fact that the objects of nature are often symmetrical. Rather, we wish to examine some of the even more remarkable symmetries of the universe—the symmetries that exist in the basic laws themselves which govern the operation of the physical world.

Richard Feynman 1963

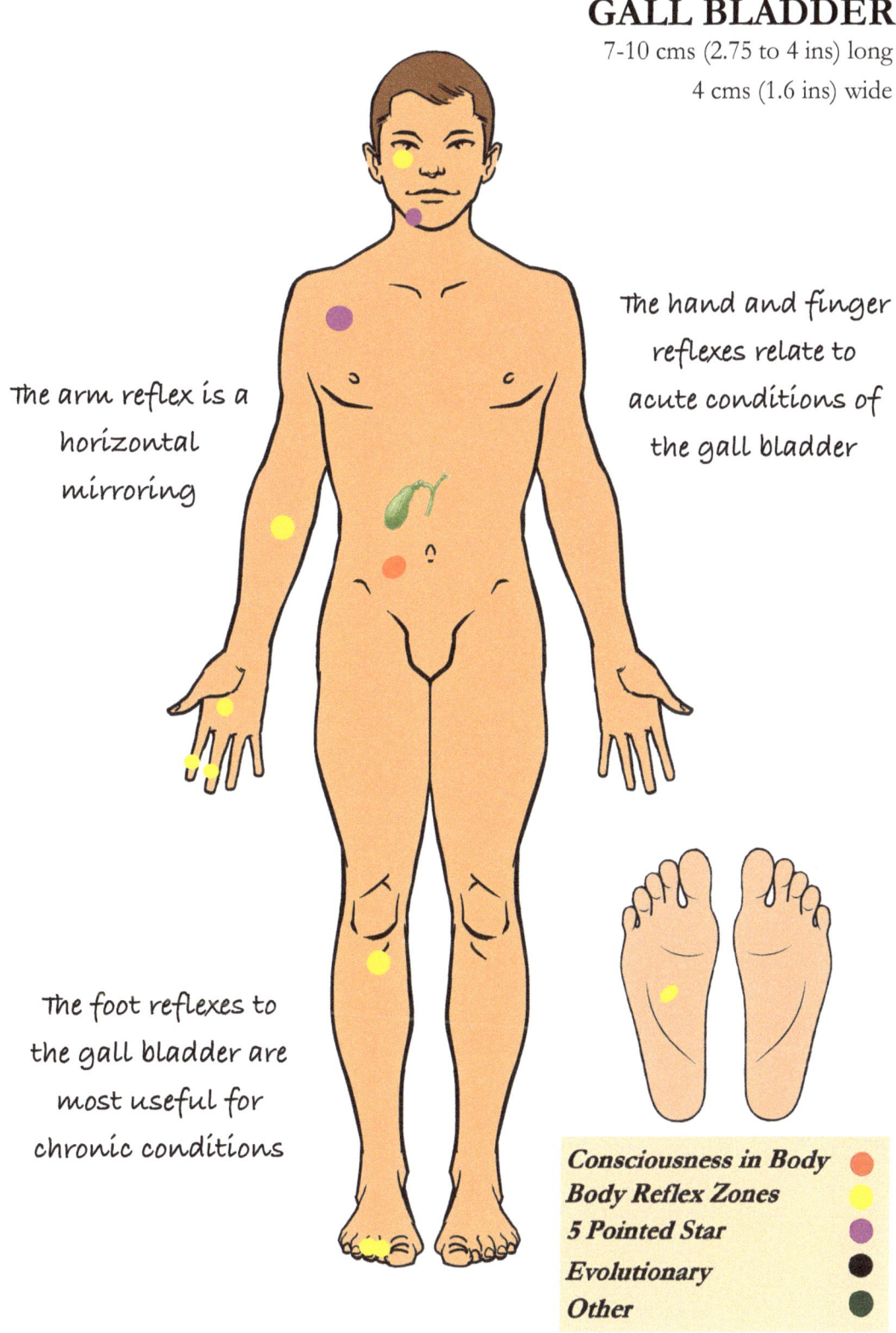

Gall Bladder Treatment

The gall bladder sits tucked beneath the liver and stores bile. When full, it is the size of a small pear. The bile aids in the breakdown of fats. Problems with it can give rise to incomplete digestion, gas production in the intestines, headaches and eye strain. Gallstones are another common problem that can create severe pain in the right shoulder.

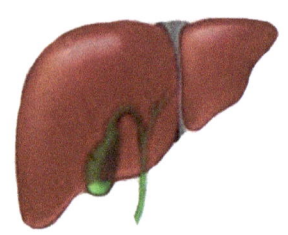

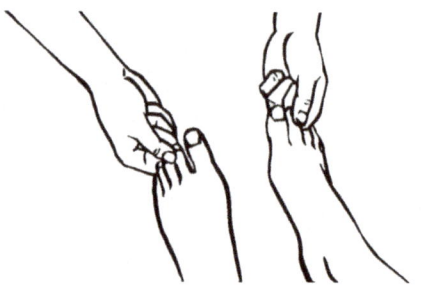

Begin by working the first joint on the second and third toes. Squeeze and stretch the toes in a milking action until any tension or pain diminishes and the energy flows more freely.

Working the first toes has an effect on the ducts from the liver and gall bladder, whilst working the third toe can have a more direct action on the gall bladder itself. The joints of the left toes are mirror reflexes.

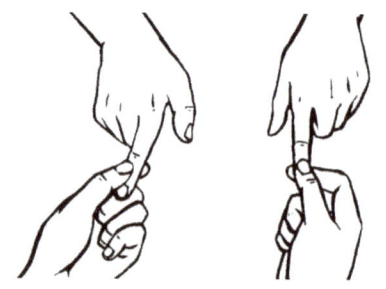

Repeat on the first joints of the forefinger and middle finger.

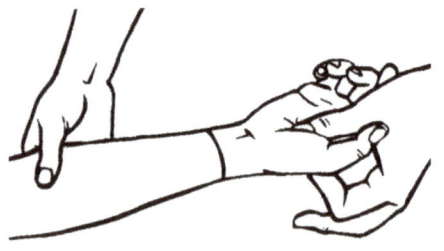

Then with the thumbs work into tender areas in the tendon interspace between the thumb and forefinger whilst alternately stimulating the reflex just below the elbow. The gall bladder is a relatively large organ so stimulation of this reflex should cover an equivalent proportional area on the arm.

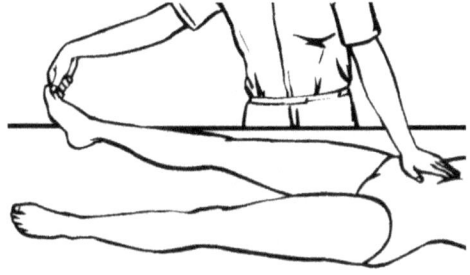

Connect the reflexes on the toes to the gall bladder which is approximately 1 inch or 2.5 cms above the navel and 2 inches or 5 cms towards the outside of the body. Stimulate this area and the toe joints alternately then wait for energetic coherence. As this technique is done over the gall bladder, apart from feeling energy you may also hear gurgling as it drains.

Then leaving the upper hand over the gall bladder, move the lower hand up to reflex just below the knee. Stimulate alternately.

Then, if required, repeat the last three techniques on the other side of the body to affect the mirror reflexes.

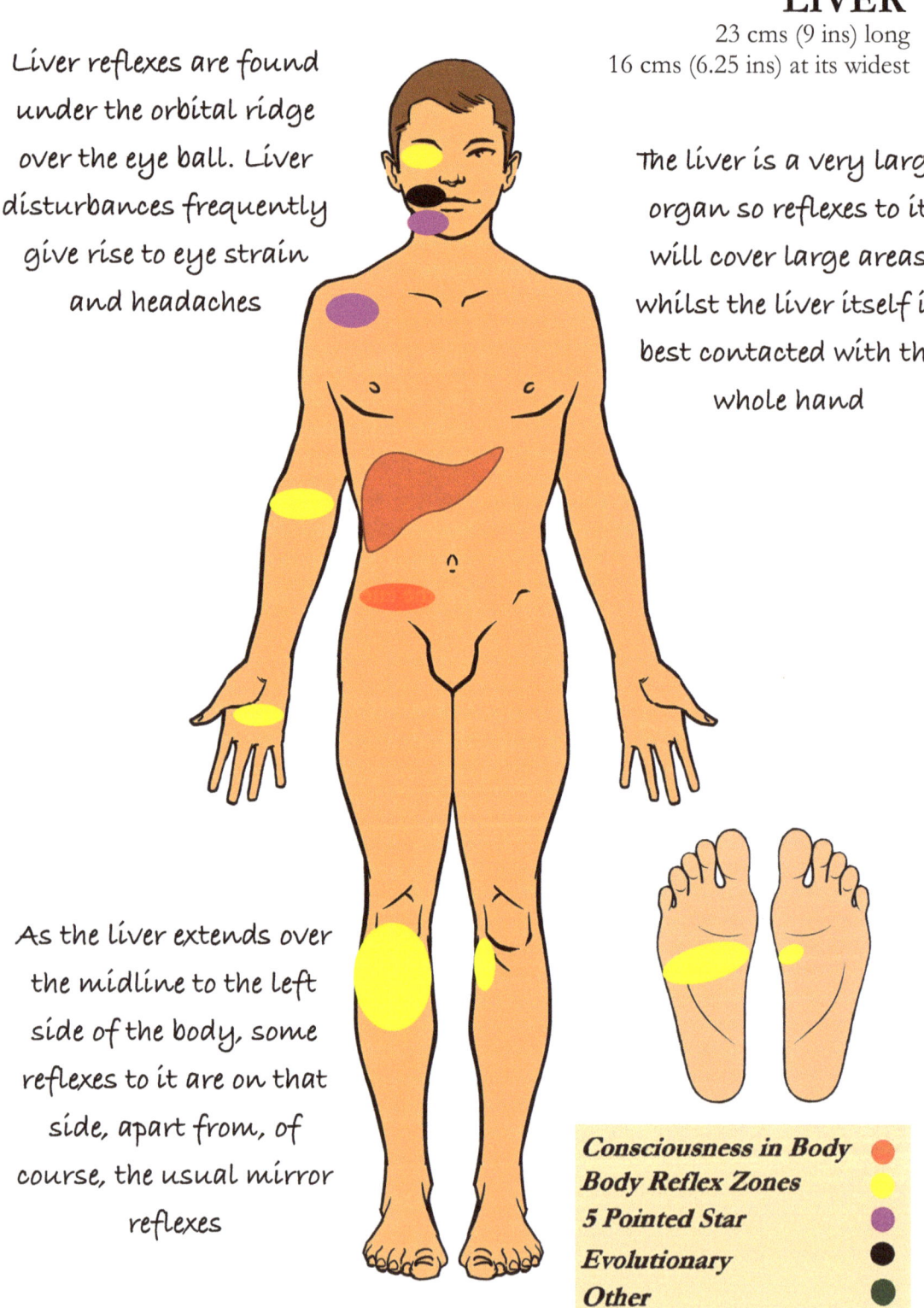

LIVER
23 cms (9 ins) long
16 cms (6.25 ins) at its widest

Liver reflexes are found under the orbital ridge over the eye ball. Liver disturbances frequently give rise to eye strain and headaches

The liver is a very large organ so reflexes to it will cover large areas whilst the liver itself is best contacted with the whole hand

As the liver extends over the midline to the left side of the body, some reflexes to it are on that side, apart from, of course, the usual mirror reflexes

Consciousness in Body ●
Body Reflex Zones ●
5 Pointed Star ●
Evolutionary ●
Other ●

Liver Treatment

The liver is the largest organ in the body. It is a complex chemical factory that works 24 hours a day, processing virtually everything you eat, drink, breathe in or rub on your skin and that's just some of its over 500 different functions vital to life.

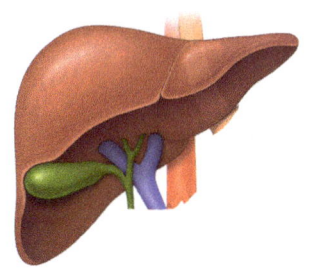

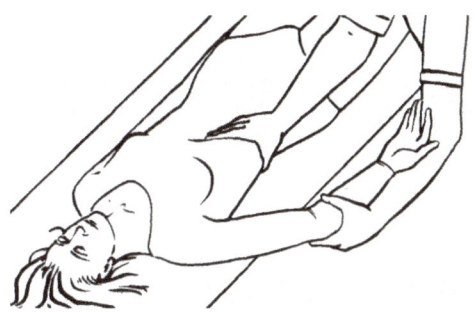

Place the right hand over the liver. Gently grasp the right elbow and place the left thumb below the crease. Stimulate these two places by rocking the body with the hand over the liver and gently squeezing the inner elbow by pressing first down and upward towards the shoulder in a smooth circular movement. Alternate these two movements for 2-3 minutes.

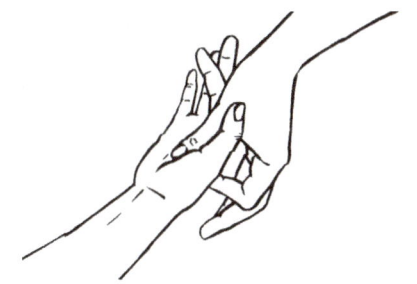

Leaving the hand over the liver, move the hand from the elbow to the client's right hand and stimulate the web between the thumb and forefinger. Alternately pulse the energy between the two contacts for 1-2 minutes and sense for coherence.

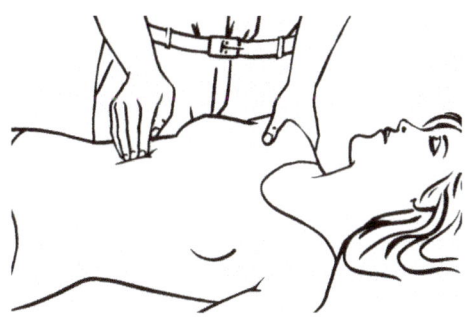

Lightly grasp the right shoulder with the left hand so that the thumb is on the liver reflexes at the shoulder. The right hand works gently over the liver area beneath the right lower ribs, using either the finger pads or the palm of the hand. Systematically work over the whole of the liver, alternating the liver contacts with a gentle stimulation of the shoulder. Then hold the hand palm down over the liver whilst maintaining the shoulder contact and listen for energetic coherence.

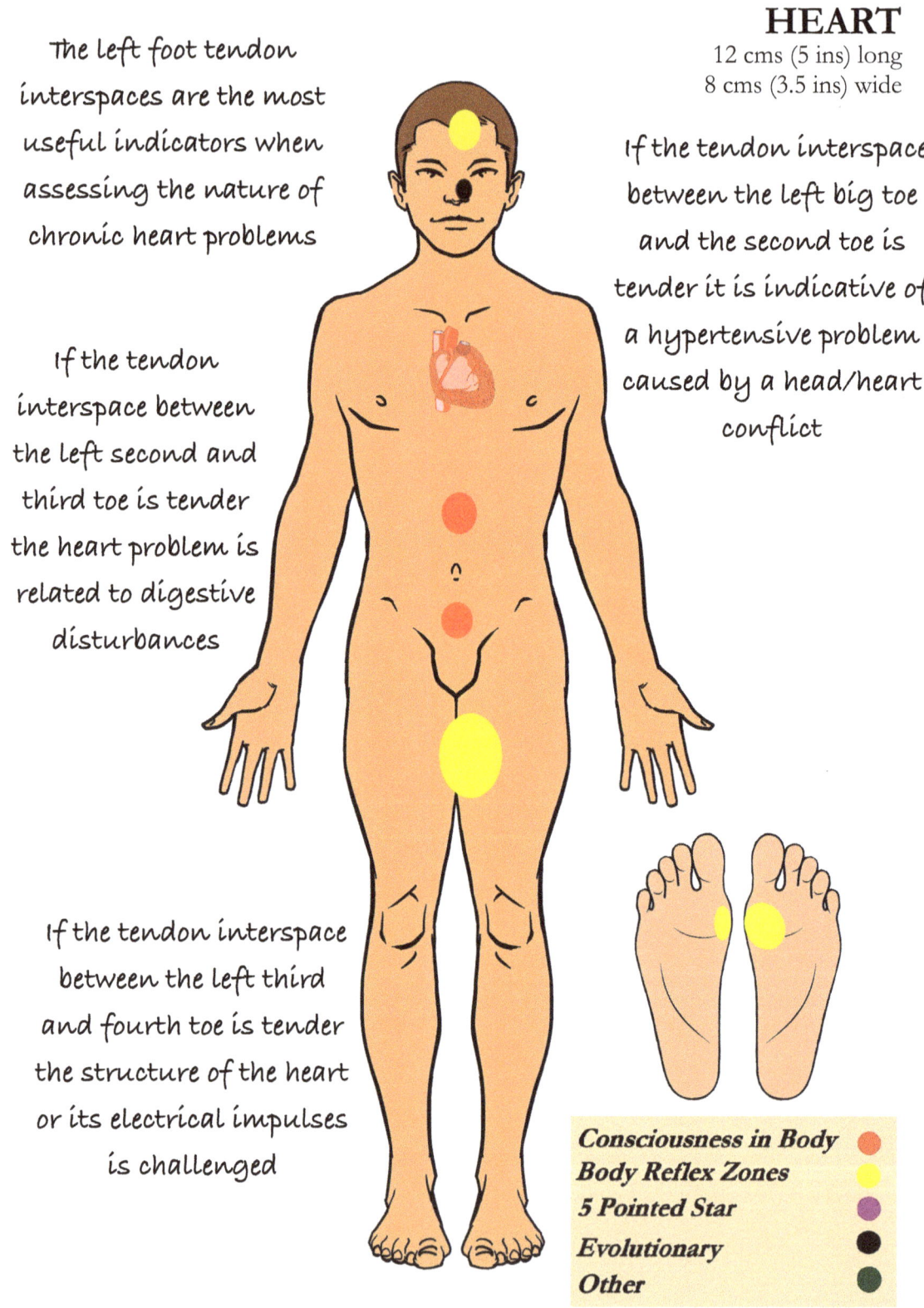

HEART
12 cms (5 ins) long
8 cms (3.5 ins) wide

The left foot tendon interspaces are the most useful indicators when assessing the nature of chronic heart problems

If the tendon interspace between the left big toe and the second toe is tender it is indicative of a hypertensive problem caused by a head/heart conflict

If the tendon interspace between the left second and third toe is tender the heart problem is related to digestive disturbances

If the tendon interspace between the left third and fourth toe is tender the structure of the heart or its electrical impulses is challenged

Consciousness in Body ●
Body Reflex Zones ●
5 Pointed Star ●
Evolutionary ●
Other ●

Heart Treatment

Your heart beats about 100,000 times each day and does the most physical work of any muscle in the body in a lifetime. It has its own electrical impulse and creates the biggest electrical field in the body. The heart can be affected by structural anomalies, diet, stress, lifestyle and emotions.

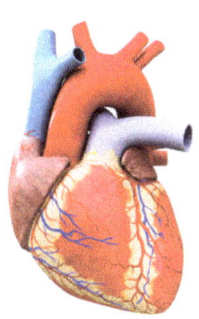

The forefingers and the second toes have a very direct influence on the heart. A very simple general heart treatment would involve stimulating these fingers and toes whilst resting the hand over the heart and gently rocking the chest to pulse the energy between the two places (see p. 96-98).

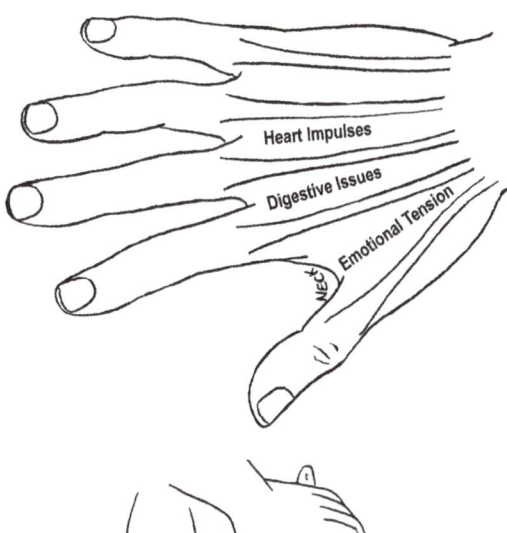

Whilst any of the heart reflexes on the chart opposite can be used in the treatment heart problems it is important to understand that most heart conditions have indirect or peripheral causative factors. The two primary factors are emotional stress and digestive issues. Of course, it is also true that the structure of the heart and the rhythmic impulse behind its beat are also significant.

To establish the most significant factor when assessing an acute heart problem, check the tendon interspaces between the thumb and first three fingers of the left hand for tenderness.

All three tendon interspaces should be treated but the most tender area should be treated for longer.

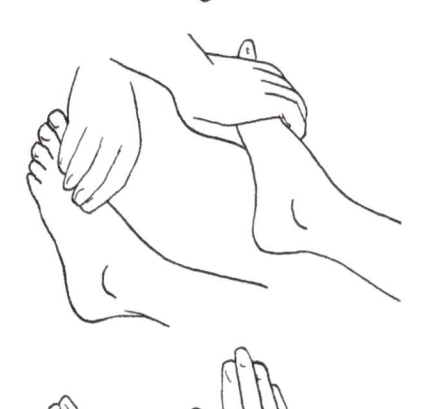

Stimulate the tendon interspaces on the feet and then the hands by working into the areas with the pads of the fingers as shown. Simultaneously work the feet, then the hands. This can most comfortably be achieved by crossing the arms.

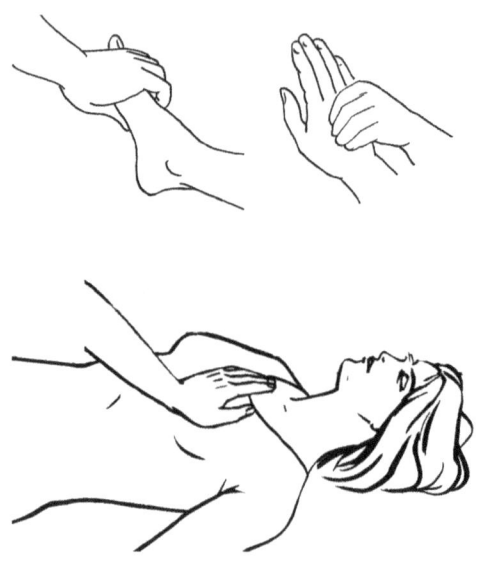

Then standing on the client's right side alternately work the tendon interspaces of the right hand and foot.

Now place the palm of the left hand over the sternum. Stimulate the tendon interspaces on the right foot, alternating with a gentle rocking of the sternum. Repeat this alternating stimulation in both places for 2-3 minutes. For ease of application the leg can be bent when connecting foot and chest.

Then leaving the left hand on the sternum work the tendon interspace on the client's right hand. Once again alternately stimulate both places for 2-3 minutes.

Stop and feel for energetic coherence after each technique.

Repeat on the other side of the body using the right hand on the sternum.

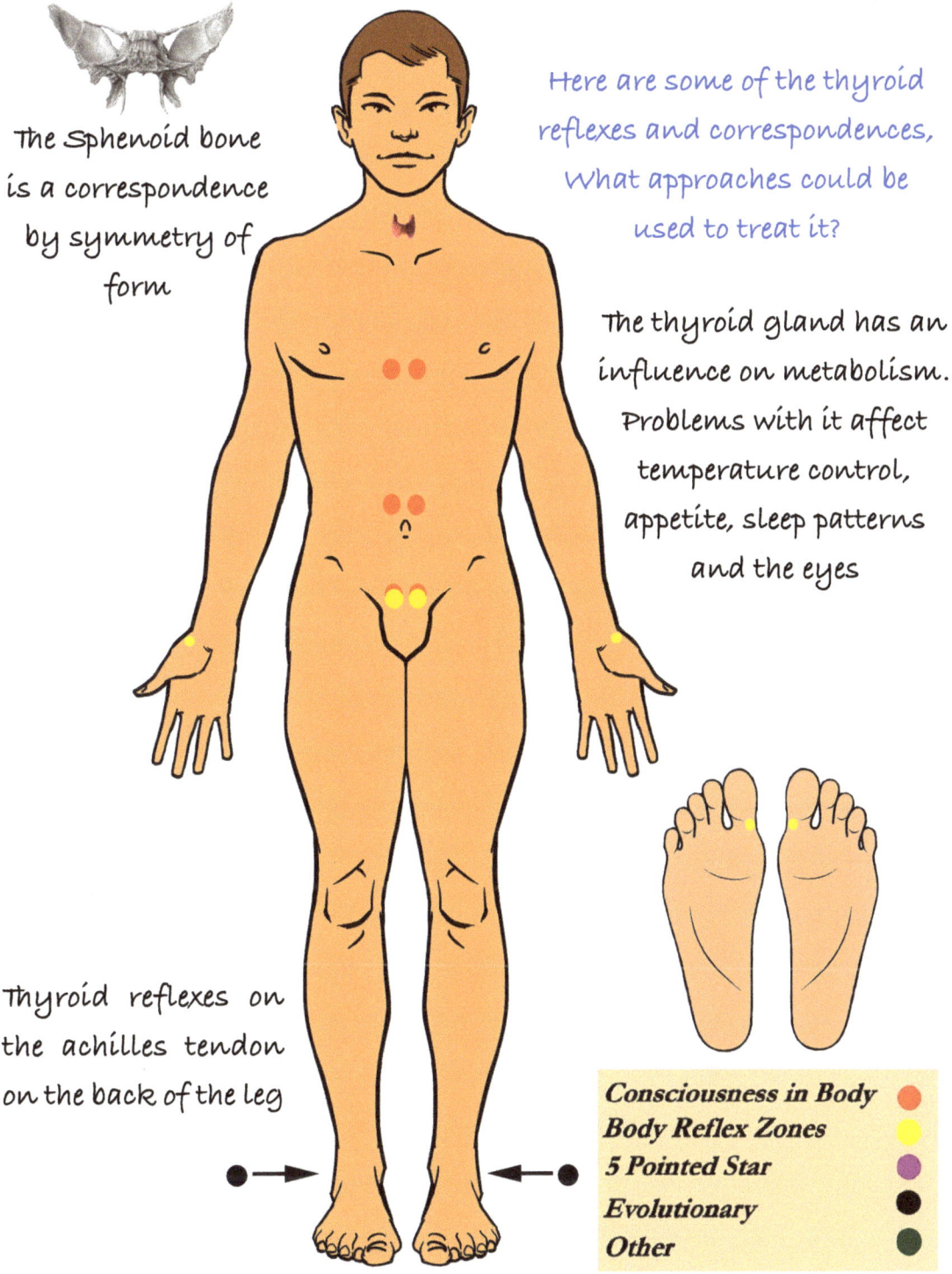

Spinal Correspondences

The spine protects your spinal cord, supports the body's weight and facilitates the movement and flexibility of the upper body.

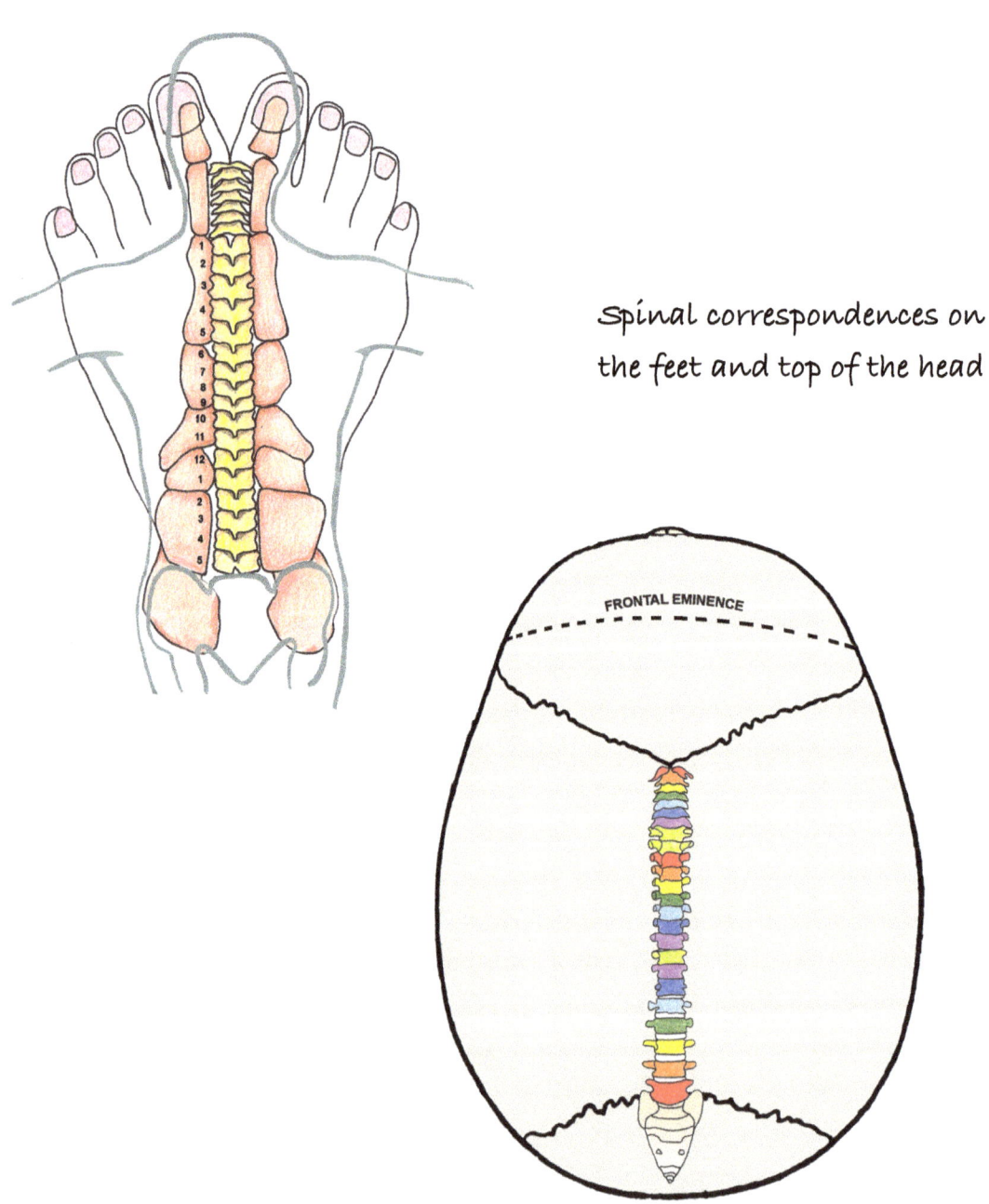

Spinal correspondences on the feet and top of the head

Vertebral Correspondences

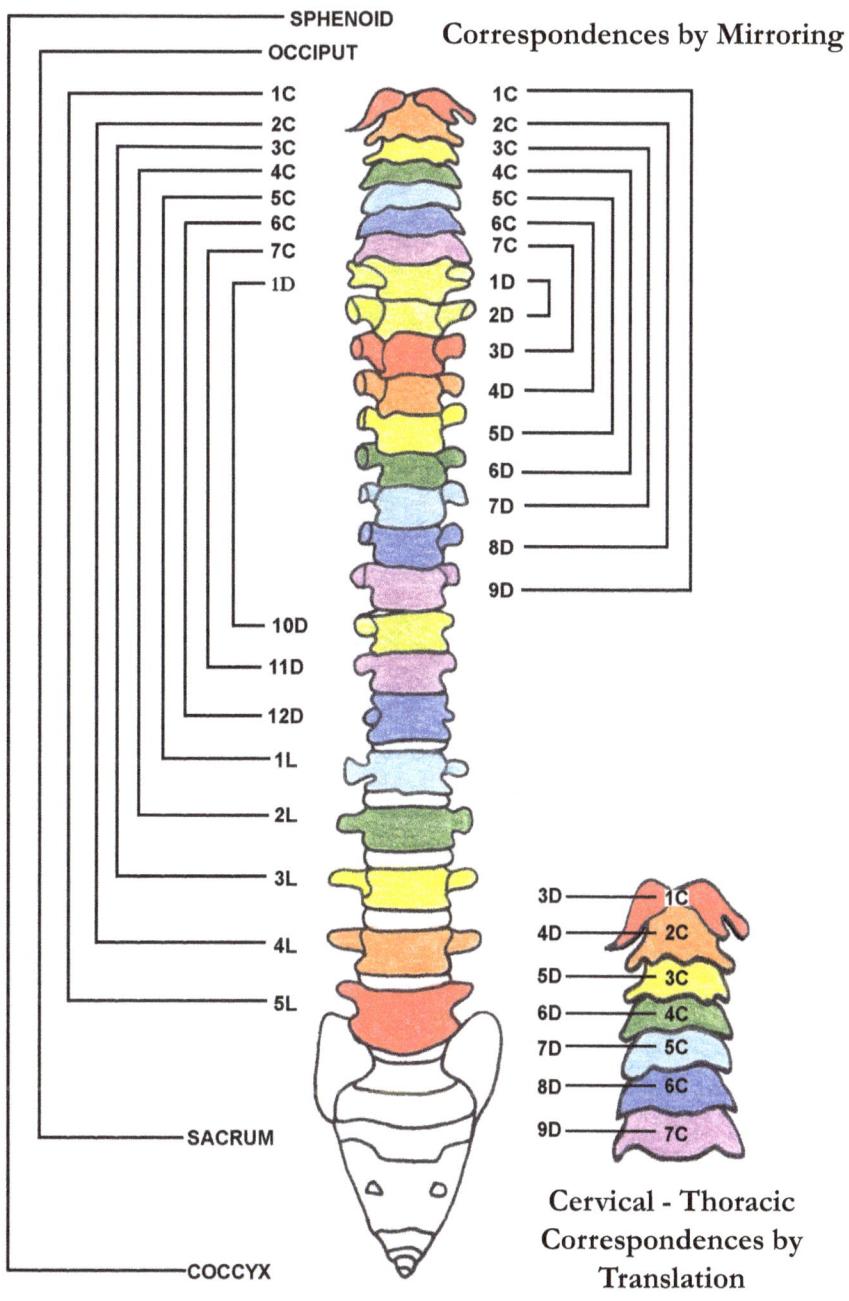

N.B. The colour coding does not apply to the upper right side mirrored cervical/thoracic vertebral correspondences.

Pain and soreness over a vertebra can be caused by a huge range of issues such as position, muscle tension, injury and nerve compression.

Pain in the lumbar spine will often be accompanied by discomfort in the neck. This is because a problem with any vertebra will tend to create problems in other related vertebrae through all the various correspondences in the vertebral column.

The chart and tables show both the mirrored and translated reflex relationships.

TRANSLATION AND MIRROR REFLEXES →

C1	D3	D9	L5
C2	D4	D8	L4
C3	D5	D7	L3
C4	D6	D6	L2
C5	D7	D5	L1
C6	D8	D4	T12
C7	D9	D3	T11

TRANSLATION REFLEXES ↓

C1	C2	C3	C4	C5	C6	C7	D1
D2	D3	D4	D5	D6	D7	D8	D9
D10	D11	D12	L1	L2	L3	L4	L5

The cervical vertebrae can translate into the thoracic spine. They also mirror into the thoracic and lumbar spine. The cervical vertebrae begin as a translation at D3 because D1 and D2 have a strong mirror relationship.

Yet another way of looking at the spinal relationships is to see that there are 24 vertebrae in total which gives 3 sets of 8 vertebrae. If we translate the first 8 vertebrae into the second we get for example C1 in harmonic resonance with D2 and when we translate C1 into the third set of 8 we get it resonating with D10.

Spinal Treatment

Working the spinal reflexes on the foot and connecting them to the actual vertebrae is a fundamental approach to working with spinal issues.

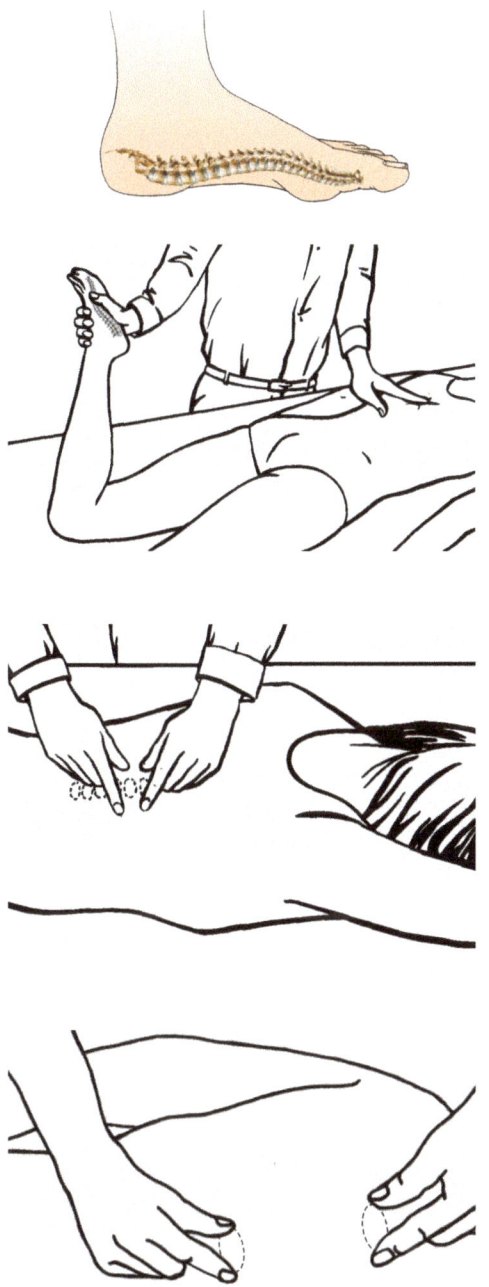

Connecting spinal foot reflexes to the spine is most comfortably done with the client face down. Bending the leg allows an easy connection from the foot reflex to the related vertebrae of the spine.

Contact the spinal reflex on the foot with your thumb and place the fingers of your other hand on the related vertebrae. Alternately stimulate both areas for 1-2 minutes and sense for energetic coherence. Repeat on the same reflex on the other foot connecting it to the same vertebrae on the back. All disturbed vertebrae can be worked in this way.

The vertebrae immediately above and below any particular vertebrae have a strong correspondence by translation. A simple treatment is to work the vertebrae above and below a problematic vertebrae.

Standing on the clients left side place your right thumb and forefinger either side of the vertebrae above the one with a problem and the thumb and forefinger of the right hand on the transverse process of the vertebrae below. Stimulate each area alternately for 1-2 minutes and then hold and sense for coherence.

Then you can connect the vertebra to the corresponding mirror or translated vertebrae as shown on the charts on the page opposite.

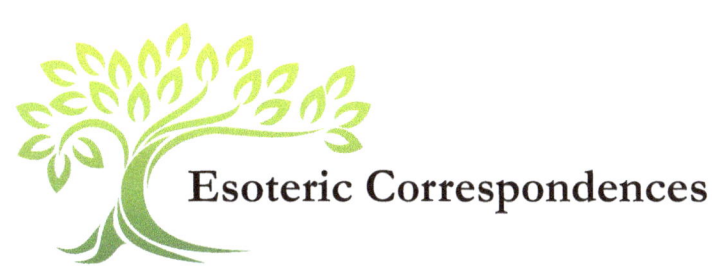

Esoteric Correspondences

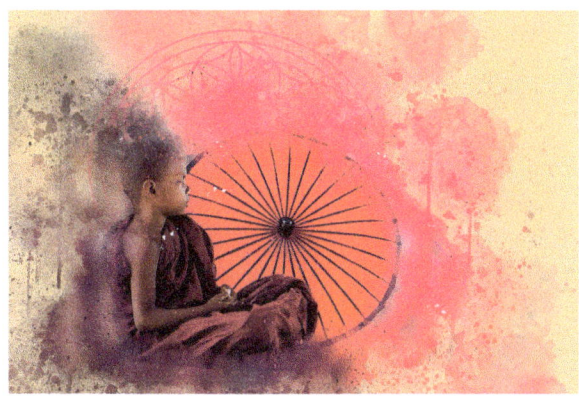

The exoteric is simply the outer observable form of something, its external facade. The esoteric is the hidden inner content and deep meaning. The exoteric view of the world is dominant in the modern Western world and is exemplified in the scientific viewpoint. The scientific world view does, of course, go deeper than the surface of things but, in that deep search that plumbs the depths of physical reality, what it loses is a perception of the meaning and significance of what it observes. Modern science is both deterministic (all things have a cause), reductive (complex things can be reduced and explained by something simpler) and materialistic (nothing exists except matter).

By contrast, the esoteric view of the world is wholistic, always looking at the big picture and the interconnectedness of things. When it looks deep inside, it is looking for the pattern, significance and meaning of what it sees. The esoteric concern is with soul and spirit rather than matter.

For the average person the challenge of living in the exoteric world is more than enough, yet for some people it does not satisfy. The cry from within these people is, "There has be more to life than just this (the exoteric)". The answer these people seek lies in spirit not matter, soul not mind. The esoteric world view and a different sense of the significance of human life is a beacon of hope to such people.

The usage of the terms esoteric and exoteric in the Western world dates back to the mid 1600s. However, their roots go much further back. In Aristotle's time (384–322 BC) the differentiation between the two words was more about the simple version for the public and the more complex and philosophical for his inner circle. According to one account, those who were deemed worthy to attend Aristotle's learned discussions were known as his esoterics', his confidants, while those who merely attended his popular evening lectures were called his 'exoterics'. Since material that is geared toward a target audience is often not as easily comprehensible to outside observers, esoteric also acquired an extended meaning of 'difficult to understand'.

A modern dictionary defines the word esoteric as:

1a : designed for or understood by the specially initiated alone

1b: requiring or exhibiting knowledge that is restricted to a small group - esoteric terminology; broadly : difficult to understand - esoteric subjects

2a: limited to a small circle engaging in esoteric pursuits : private, confidential an esoteric purpose

3: of special, rare, or unusual interest, esoteric building materials

Whereas the word exoteric, being the opposite of esoteric, means 'suitable to be imparted to the public'.[1]

By the middle ages, the idea that the esoteric related to hidden knowledge that one had to be initiated into was a dominant understanding. The concept of initiation is multi-layered but from an esoteric perspective the teaching of this particular world view needs to come from someone who knows i.e. not just someone who knows the concepts intellectually but who embodies them in their whole life. This person is a keeper or carrier of the secret. When you study with them, it is their embodiment of the esoteric that is transmitted, via a kind of deep unconscious osmosis, rather than just their words and ideas. At a later stage, there is often an initiation ceremony. That ceremonial process is more an open acknowledgement of the progress the student has already made rather than any kind of immediate transmission of either knowledge or power during the ceremony itself.

Esoteric knowledge was also taught in secret because the internal unfoldment of the esoteric is like a fragile flower that can easily be damaged before it has come to full bloom and born fruit. This is why, in his Sermon on the Mount, Jesus says, "Neither caste ye your pearls before swine, lest they trample them under their feet, and turn and tear you in pieces", meaning that sharing something that is so precious and sacred with people who have no respect or appreciation for it is dangerous because they, at they very least, will scorn and belittle it and some will go so far as to persecute you.

---

1. https://www.merriam-webster.com/dictionary/esoteric

Since the middle of first millennium, the dominance of orthodox religion, coupled with the later emergence of the scientific world view during the last 350 years of the second millennium, have formed the basis of the exoteric in the Western world. Part of the power of orthodox religion and the scientific world view are that they are self-referencing and totally invalidate all other positions or world views, under both the guise and pretence that these two offer mankind some hope of salvation either by God or the miracles of science, and therefore any opposite position or differing world view is denounced as either the work of the Devil or pseudo-scientific quackery. So, it is no surprise then that by the mid 1500s the teaching of an esoteric perspective on the world went underground and was taught in secret. It needed to be in secret to escape religious persecution and later on to avoid scientific ridicule. From the esoteric perspective, personal experience is all important and is the basis of an inner personal authority. Whereas in the exoteric all personal authority is given over to external figures such as members of the clergy or the high priests of science.

> "Scientific knowledge not only enjoys universal esteem but, in the eyes of modern man, counts as the only intellectual and spiritual authority".
> *The Undiscovered Self* - Carl G. Jung - 1957

In ancient Greece and Egypt the whole of life was experienced from an esoteric perspective and this is still true of many indigenous peoples today. You could say that in these cultures, that it was an open secret.

Esoteric Healing—Exoteric Therapy

Whether openly acknowledged or not, a great many modern therapies have their roots in esoteric concepts of healing that go back to ancient Greece and Egypt, concepts that were still prevalent in the middle ages in Europe. In about 1010AD Avicenna wrote a "Cannon of Medicine". This canon was the basis of medical practice in Europe until the late 1700s. Avicenna was actually the Persian, Ibn Sina (980-1037). He drew heavily on the original teachings of Hippocrates (c. 460 – c. 370 BC) and Galen (129 AD – c. 200/c. 216) whose medical treatises had been translated into Arabic and were widely available in the Islamic world.

The basis of what Avicenna taught, concerned:

1. The Nature of the human being as a Whole

2. The Constitution

3. The Breath as Energy

4. The Elements (Earth, Air, Fire and Water)

> "It is far more important to know what person the disease has than what disease the person has".
>
> Hippocrates

All of these principles would be familiar to practitioners of many current systems of alternative and complementary therapy.

In the 18th and 19th centuries these principles continued to inform the practice of so called empirical medicine. This form of medicine was just as dominant, if not more so, than the practice of allopathic medicine. These empirical approaches, such as herbalism, homoeopathy, mesmerism, naturopathy and osteopathy, worked in co-operation with nature and considered the life force an intrinsic aspect of their work. These and many other therapies based upon the stimulation and balance of the vital life force were in significant decline by the late 1920s, due largely to the influence of 'Flexner's Medical Education in the United States and Canada: A Report to the Carnegie Foundation for the Advancement of Teaching (1910)'. However, by the late 1960s with the emergence of the human potential movement, a new era of interest in healing work began and the practice of empirical medicine surged under the new title of 'Alternative and Complementary Medicine'. Since the 1980s, the modern Western scientific world view has gradually become pervasive in both the teaching and practice of alternative and complementary therapy. Most therapies have been caught up in issues related to defining scope of practice, proving their efficacy scientifically and dealing with general legislative issues. Therapies have, in a sense, become more and more exoteric losing the connection to the roots of their creation which lie in the esoteric world view.

The greatest difference between the therapists in our modern era and healers in the ancient world is that modern therapy is simply a career choice based upon exoteric considerations whereas in the ancient world it was a calling—an esoteric process. A person was called by the gods to become a healer. Even in our modern world some people who become therapists are really healers. They have answered a calling. A calling that comes from deep within. Equally, there are many people who call themselves healers who are really therapists.

One might ask what need is there for an understanding and acknowledgement of the esoteric within modern therapies as the exoteric therapeutic approach is admirably suited to most of the types of physical and emotional problems that beset patients. Yet in reality, there are many problems and life issues that cannot be easily addressed via an exoteric approach. Broadly speaking, these are problems of the deep psyche and soul, such issues can have a profound effect on the physical and emotional experience of patients. These types of problems can arise in anyone regardless of whether or not they are guided by an exoteric world view upon life or live with an esoteric perspective. These type of problems are not amenable to treatment via exoteric therapeutic approaches.

One of the key differences between the exoteric and esoteric approach to health is choice. An exoteric approach to therapy gives repeatable results and can be tested. Its goal is to cure. An esoteric approach to healing acknowledges that both health and illness are choices. Esoteric healing allows a client to choose whether or not to be healed and the process cannot be tested. Its goal is to heal. Healing means the client both gains insight into the nature of the challenge they are facing and gives them the ability to consciously choose their path, wherever it may lead. When you just analyse the outer form of a therapy, in terms of its theories and techniques, you miss the essence which is hidden and esoteric.

In an exoteric approach the skill of the practitioner and their ability to apply the technique of their chosen therapeutic modality is all important. In esoteric healing, the technique and skill of the practitioner is secondary. Who the practitioner is, the level of their own personal development is all that matters, their healing presence. An older term for this was the doctor's bedside manner.

Doctors and exoteric therapists have clients. Esoteric healers have patients (patience). This, of course, is the exact opposite of the way things are usually expressed in modern Western medicine. In many countries it is generally considered inappropriate for therapists and healers to refer to the people they work with as patients, this term being arrogated to the medical profession. However, the original derivation of the term patient lay in the fact that since ancient times, before the advent of molecular medicine, natural healing took time. Even today if you take a heavy fall and bruise your body the tissues will heal, the bruising appear and disperse in its own time. You just have to be patient.

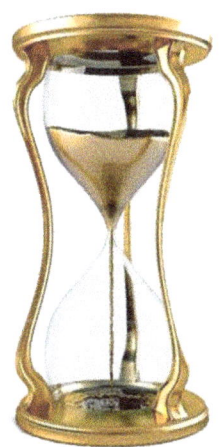

"Healing is a matter of time, but it is sometimes a matter of opportunity".
Precepts chapter 1 - Hippocrates

Beneath the health care practices of today lie buried an esoteric knowledge that has been forgotten or dismissed yet has a potency to restore health to the individual at each level of being.

In our modern era people seeking healing go to a therapist. They enter a dedicated therapeutic space (treatment room) where they receive advice as well as other types of direct intervention such as physical manipulation to resolve their problems. This is a simple exoteric process.

In ancient Egypt and Greece healing took place in temples dedicated to the god Asclepius and healing took place through a process called temple sleep. A person needing healing visited a temple where, having shed their everyday clothing and cleansed their body, they entered into the inner sanctum where they would simply lie down on a plinth and go to sleep. Their understanding was that during that deep temple sleep the gods would appear in a dream and heal them, either directly or through giving advice on what they needed to do to regain their health.

A modern esoteric approach consciously acknowledges that the treatment room is a temple of healing. The bodywork table is the plinth and the deep insights that emerge from the altered states of consciousness that patients experience as a hidden aspect of conscious energetic touch is the temple sleep.

A BODYWORK TABLE

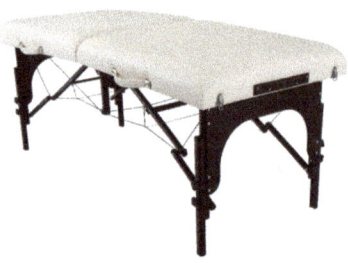

add a dark cover and it becomes

AN ALTAR

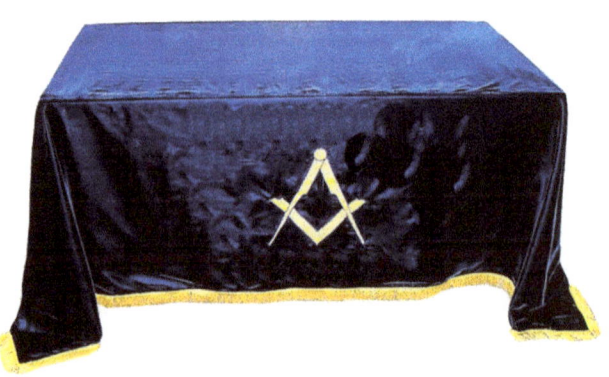

Healing as Transformation

The esoteric perspective on healing is fundamentally concerned with the transformation of being. Transformation is a thread that runs through many ancient esoteric practices, a prime example being alchemy where it is often referred to as the transformation of base metal into gold, which understood psychologically, is the transformation of your character and personality. Transformation is essentially the process of rising above one's nature and its limitations (created by inheritance, family and education) and becoming a new man or woman. This transformational process can be described in many ways. In ancient Greece, one of the most significant was through the understanding of the role of mathematics in relation to human life. This concept dates back to Pythagoras (500BC) and his followers. Pythagorean thought was dominated by the belief that numbers and mathematics were the key to understanding the true nature of things. Numbers were representative of the principle of a divine order in the Universe. They held that the study of philosophy and mathematics constituted a moral basis for living one's life. Indeed, the word philosophy (love of wisdom) and mathematics (that which is learned) are said to have been created by Pythagoras.

Mathematics of Consciousness

In the theoretical sections of this book we explored the significance of geometry on Holonomic Reflexology, but from an esoteric perspective, mathematics is equally important.

The Pythagoreans believed that a greater force or archetype lay behind and worked through the use of numbers. They believed the simple act of counting 1, 2, 3, 4, 5, 6 held great hidden inner or esoteric significance as the numbers themselves represent something much deeper - nothing less than a model of human consciousness. These numbers can also be represented by a set of geometric shapes beginning with a point, a line, a triangle, a square and 5 and 6 pointed stars.

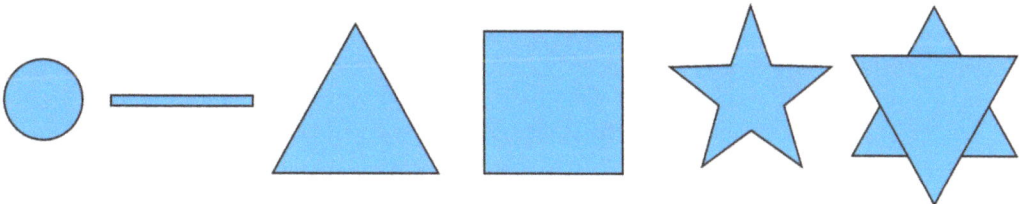

The number 1, or a point, signifies that the human being begins as single point of consciousness in the cosmos, a monad or unity. Birth and entering the larger physical world is the beginning of active awareness and consciousness. It is no small thing to maintain awareness and consciousness throughout life. Many spiritual traditions speak of human beings as being prone to 'fall asleep' as they grow and mature, and that the ability to maintain true, single pointed consciousness and awareness throughout one's life is a great achievement.

In early infancy, the human being is represented by the number 2, or the polarity of a line, which, of course, has two ends, which represent the beginning of the duality of conscious experience. At this stage human consciousnesss is dyadic. The shift from 1 to 2 is an automatic process. In dyadic consciousness man thinks and experiences the world as pairs of opposites. All his thoughts, feelings, sensations and emotions can be divided into positive and negative, yes and no, right and wrong, black and white. At this level, thought opposes feeling and emotion.

In this relatively high energy state, these polarities exchange places frequently and seemingly randomly. It is extremely difficult to use one's will to assert control over these opposites as the whole organism functions in a random and mechanical fashion. Over time, all living systems have a tendency to reach a particular balance or state of equilibrium and so, after a time, the energy of polarity becomes exhausted and the tension between the opposing states decreases, leading to a certain kind of balance but one lacking in vitality. This is a mechanical balance that lacks any real sense of conscious control. A person at this stage can often feel paralysed and stuck. What is needed is a shift or a step up in consciousness.

The state of polarity is transformed into a triad or trinity through the addition of a neutral organising centre at a higher frequency or level of consciousness. The state of consciousness represented by the number 3, or a trinity, has a great deal of energy in it. This new state resolves the stagnation that is often a part of the dualistic state of consciousness by giving a new perspective or viewpoint. It is no longer yes or no but by rising to a higher level, the two polarities, the two sides of dyadic consciousness, can be perceived all at once as no longer two but simply as the two sides of the same coin, or two aspects of the same thing. This new kind of perception liberates all the energy that was stuck in the stagnant dyadic state.

The triadic state of consciousness (positive, negative and neutral) is a kind of 3 in 1 or unity that has a much higher level of energy than the dyadic state even at its most vibrant. However, once again over time, a state of stable equilibrium begins to emerge as all three points of the triangle gradually assume equal potency and the whole organism again becomes too stable and the level of vitality within it begins to drop. At this stage, another shift of consciousness is required in which a new organising centre must be found, or created at a higher frequency, to once more take the organism back into a state of dynamism.

What emerges now is the number 4, the tetrad or quaternity commonly represented by the square. Once again enormous amounts of energy are liberated and profound transformation is possible.

The square and its division by an internal cross represents a fundamental coordinate system for time and space, the microcosm and the macrocosm. The tetrad is the basis for many models of the world we experience: four elements (air, fire, water, earth), four seasons (winter, spring, summer, autumn), four directions (north, east, south, west), four Evangelists (Matthew, Mark, Luke, John), four ancient ages (gold, silver, bronze, iron), the four rivers of the paradise and, as Carl Jung proposed, the four can also be represented by the processes of sensing, feeling, thinking and intuition.

In geometry, a fourth point can transform a two-dimensional triangle into a figure with depth and volume; the tetrahedron. Any three-dimensional structure can be viewed in four ways: as points, lines, areas, and volumes, or as corners, edges, faces, and from the centre outward.

This shift from human development expressed in terms of two dimensional plane structures (point, line, surface) to three dimensional structures is of extraordinary significance, because it is only when man has reached the level of development symbolised by three dimensional structures that he or she can be said to have become truly human, fully self-conscious and self-aware.

Any system of four elements has the potential to transform itself. As such, a four element system represents both being and becoming. To make bread requires four basic elements flour, yeast, water and fire. The balance and interaction of these four elements can be modulated in many different ways. Some will produce better bread than others. In this example, the essential actions within the process are blending, activating, transforming and fixing. The varied elements within a tetrad represent its being and all the possible interactions within it represent becoming or transformation. The tetrad shown, as either the cross within the square, or in three dimensions as the tetrahedron, implies the sense of directionality and goal orientation. Within the tetrad there is both a motivation to achieve something and the instruments with which to achieve that goal.

The expression of being and becoming in the tetrad therefore follows a certain internal orderliness or lawfulness, in terms of the interaction of any components within it, necessary for the achievement of a particular goal. Behind all the possible processes and degrees of interaction lie both reason and cause.

The level of vitality in all the possible interactions within the tetrad can decrease over time and a stable equilibrium become manifest. As before, this stability can feel internally like stagnation so, yet again, there is the need for a shift to a higher level of organisation.

With the addition of a new organising centre, man at number 4, governed by the tetrad or quaternity moves on to number 5, the pentad, often symbolised by the 5 pointed star, the symbol of the movement of consciousness inward and upward.

In the first phase of the development of human consciousness as represented by the 5 pointed star the manifestation of wilful intent is profound. Decisions can be made and carried through in a way never before possible. In ancient times, the 5 pointed star represented man's dominion over the four elements of the natural world (air, fire, water and earth). That dominion was achieved through an act of will. Another aspect that emerges in this first phase is the sense of meaning, a meaning that becomes evident through the experience of one's potential and its manifestation through acts of will.

In the second phase, as consciousness continues to be drawn inward and upward it eventually begins to connect with something beyond the self, then the personal will that was initially so evident begins to become subordinate to transpersonal will. At this stage, a unique transformation of mind, emotion and body begins to appear, where one's whole life is lived with a nascent sense of contact with the Divine and all that this might entail. Many will never even reach this level of development, let alone move beyond it. It is expressed in the word's of Jesus's prayer "nevertheless not my will, but thine, be done."

Ultimately, a stable equilibrium at this level of development of human consciousness will inevitably appear, requiring the activation of another new organising centre of consciousness.

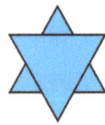
This new stage is symbolised by the number 6, the hexad, symbolised by the 6 pointed star which is also known as the Seal of Solomon the King. The number 6 is the smallest perfect number. It is the sum of 1, 2, and 3, and 6 is also divisible by each of these numbers.

In ancient Greece it was often shown by a sequence of six points. A perfectly balanced symbol.

Now the inward and upward movement of the 5 pointed star is reconciled by the movement of consciousness from above, flowing downward and outward. The 6 pointed star, represents the perfect expression of the Divine will on Earth. The numbers 1 through 4 (point, line, triangle, square) represent man's quest for personal self-development and the numbers 5 and 6 (5 and 6 pointed stars) relate to man's spiritual development moving from self-realisation to god-realisation. The 6 pointed star represents the movement of consciousness both inward and upward and downward and outward simultaneously. Consciousness at this stage always tends to stay in a state of high vitality. It does not fall into the previously mentioned states of stable or static equilibrium as it is being constantly nourished from a greater source than the self.

This model of human consciousness is a useful aid in helping to understand the level of development a patient is working with in their life. This information can offer unique insights into the kind of challenges they are facing as they work toward regaining health and well-being.

Whilst this is a hierarchical model, the manifestation of these mathematical forces or archetypes of the numbers from 1—6 do not necessarily occur in a sequential form as a developmental process. They all have the potential to be active at any time in human consciousness. Only some may be active in one's work life, whereas all may be active in another area, such as your personal life.

For example, during a single day we can be captured by polarised (2) thinking about a certain issue at work and then jump to the pentad (5), exploring how we can wilfully influence the situation which might lead us back to the trinity (3) whereby we see both sides of the problem simultaneously. This could then lead to the tetrad (4), where we sit and meditate on all the difference aspects of the problem and consider which elements and what type of interaction might transform the issue. Finally, this might take us to the hexad (6), where we find ultimate balance and resolution.

Esoterically, as part of a journey of transformation, this model can indeed be used as a sequential developmental process. This would be done by focusing your attention on the relevant concepts behind each number, starting with number 1 and then reflecting upon the degree to which it is active in your psyche and in what areas of your life. You would then work on your emotions and thought processes to bring that numerical archetype to a state of conscious control internally, as well as being able to express its nature in a balanced form externally. Then, before a state of stable equilibrium emerged, you would transform your consciousness through shifting your attention to the next number in the sequence and begin working on that.

All the various correspondences that are related to these numerical archetypes are a potential or *dynamis* that can be activated at any time regardless of your level of development.

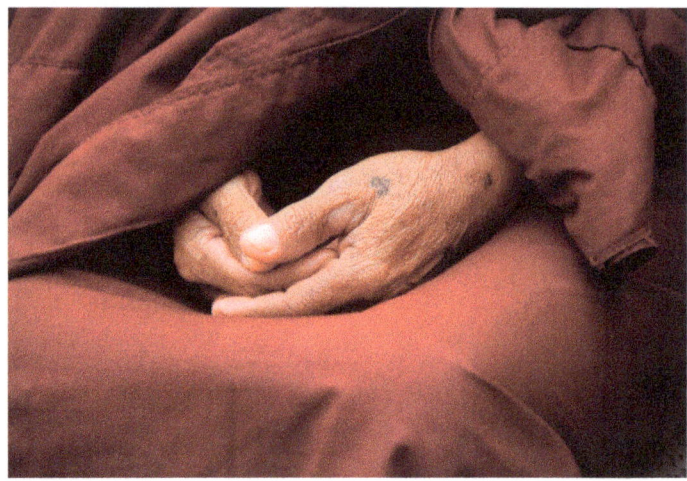

All the correspondences in the human body can be related to the numbers 1 through 6.

1. No correspondences—all is one (birth). Consciousness/energy
2. Simple polarised correspondences based upon all the various perspectives of top/bottom, front/back/left/right of the whole or part of the body.
3. Triadic correspondences such as the astrological signs and related body parts and harmonic correspondences based on 3, 6, and 9
4. Tetrad correspondences—The four natural elements.
5. Five pointed star correspondences. Evolutionary bow position.
6. Six pointed star correspondences (rebirth). Consciousness in the body. The body in consciousness. Correspondences derived from symmetry of form–the underlying pattern.

Signs and Symbols

The shapes of circle, line, triangle, and square that represent the numbers 1-4 are used in everyday life as signs. We see them used in many different ways as, for example, warning signs and to indicate speed limits. Essentially, over time these signs come to mean something to the public through general usage.

In our modern world, apart from signs, we are also used to seeing diagrams which are simplified graphics that express the essential aspects of the appearance or workings of something. A map is a diagram, rather than an exact representation of the territory.

When we consider the shape of the five and six pointed stars as representing the numbers 5 and 6, we are moving from away from the everyday realm of signs and diagrams into that of symbols. Symbols are not representative, nor is their meaning generally understood. A symbol evokes something deeper. Symbols are beyond simple logic. Pondering upon the significance of a symbol can lead to a breakthrough in perception that allows the world to be experienced in new ways. Symbols are, in essence, mysterious and can be a doorway to transcendence and transformation.

> "Thus a word or an image is symbolic when it implies something more than its obvious and immediate meaning. It has a wider 'unconscious' aspect that is never precisely defined or fully explained. Nor can one hope to define or explain it. As the mind explores the symbol, it is led to ideas that lie beyond the grasp of reason".
> *Man and his Symbols* - Carl Jung - 1964

Energy and the 5 and 6 Pointed Stars

The esoteric perspective on life is deeply related to the symbolic significance of the numbers 5 and 6 but before we explore the nature the 5 and 6 pointed stars and the correspondences that they create it is important to outline the relationship of these two stars in relation to the life energy.

In a very general sense, there is a direction of flow of life energy in the human being. It moves longitudinally up and down, pulsates from the centre out to the periphery and back, as well as moving in spirals. Both of these symbols appear in the energy body of the human being, not so much as flows of energy, but more as vibrating energetic forms. The quality of conscious represented by these two symbols is so powerful that some of the particles (or waves) of energy become more strongly attracted and so the energy begins to behave more like a solid appearing in more or less fixed positions within the overall flow of the life energy.

Within the 5 pointed star there is some general movement of consciousness and energy upward, yet that flow is not, in anyway, as fast as that of the general movement in the energy body. When we consider the energetic aspect of the 6 pointed star we are dealing with an even higher level of consciousness that is in perfect balance, a balance that creates an inherent stability.

When interacting with the 5 pointed star pattern, through conscious touch, it would be normal to engage with the energy with a certain directionality i.e. upward, this being consistent with the understanding of the significance of this form in terms of the transformation of human consciousness. You would, in effect, be temporarily creating an increase in the speed of movement of the energy through this vibrating form in the direction of your intent. This movement would help to inform the transformation of consciousness as well as intensifying the action of the physical correspondences represented by the pattern.

When interacting with the 6 pointed star, the focus is on the inherent stability and structure of the star and the balance between its upper and lower aspects. Holding these attributes in your consciousness, as an intent, is most important.

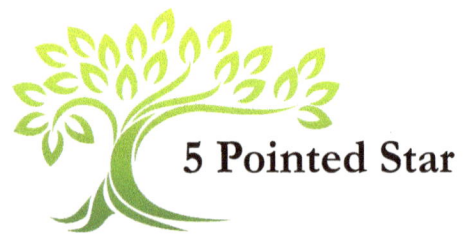

5 Pointed Star

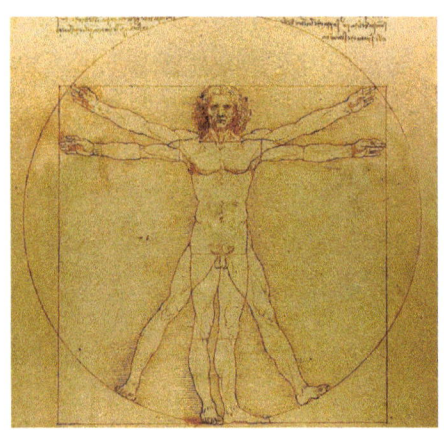

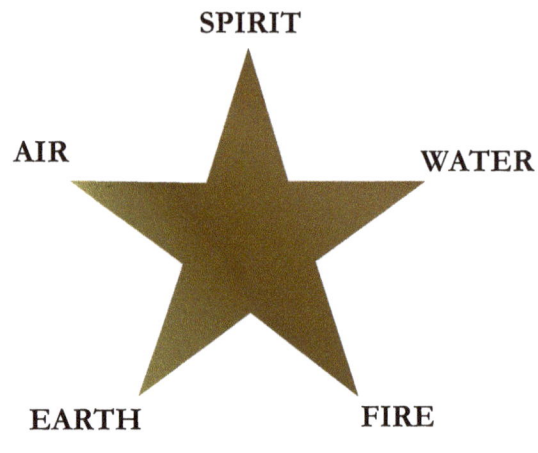

Leonardo Da Vinci's Vitruvian man is considered by some to symbolise the perfected human—God's likeness in human form through the principle of As Above, So Below. The 5 pointed star represents the stars in the heavens—the macrocosm, being reflected here on earth in the human body—the microcosm. It represents the four limbs controlled by head (mind). It is also seen as a depiction of spirit presiding over the four natural elements of Air, Fire, Water and Earth.

In ancient Greece this form was associated with health and they referred to the pentagram as a representation of Ὑγιεία – Hygieia, who was one of the daughters of Asclepius. She was considered one of the goddesses of health. We still acknowledge this in the modern world through the importance of hygiene for good health. The Pythagoreans labelled each of the points of the star with the first Greek letters for each of the four elements plus the first letter of ether/idea which actually spells the name Hygieia.

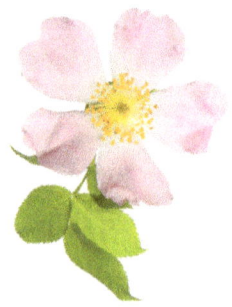

The pentagram as a symbol of the feminine principle was embodied by the dog rose. The small, five petaled roses found in the ornamentation of many Gothic cathedrals are not-so-secret 5 pointed stars.

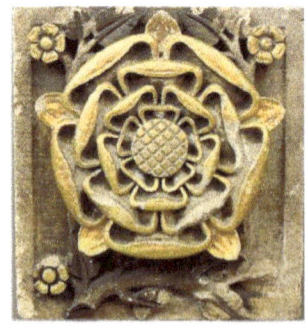

The 5 Pointed Star in Nature

The 5 pointed star is deeply imbedded in the human psyche. It is simply everywhere, in logos, advertising, magical ritual, amulets, and as a symbol of the eternal regenerative powers of nature. It is in nature that we most often see the 5 pointed star. It is, for example, present in flowers, seeds and star fishes. Cut an apple in half and there is a 5 pointed star. Look closely at a borage flower and there is a 5 pointed star.

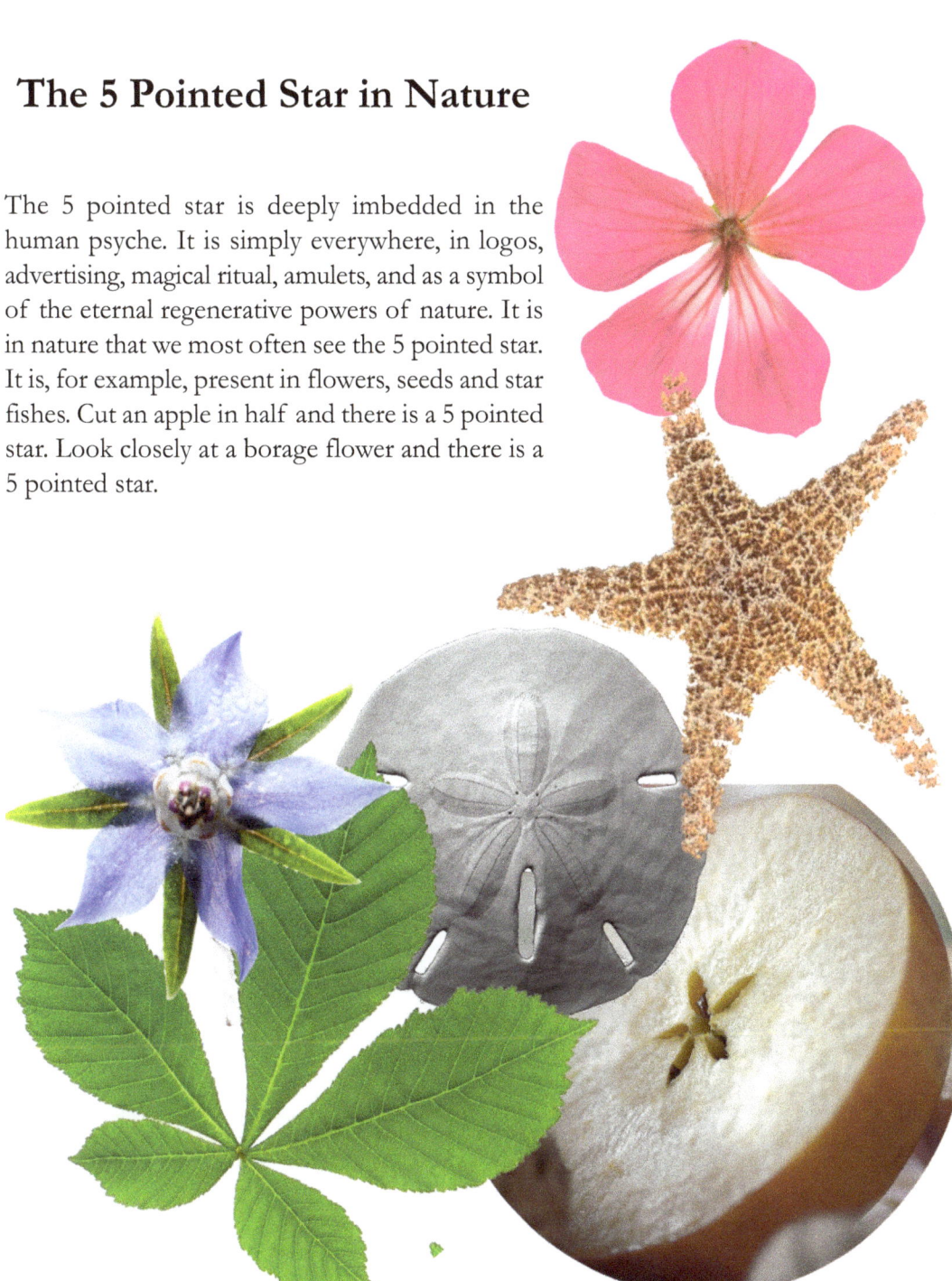

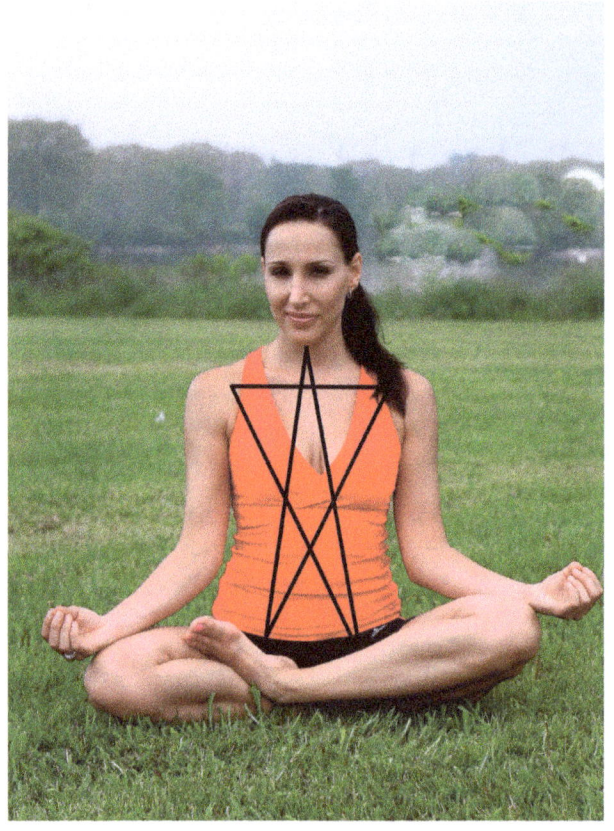

One of the geometric properties of the pentagram is that it can replicate forever smaller and larger versions of itself. The star can replicate and invert itself in its own central pentagon in an endless series. It is therefore a pattern that symbolises regeneration.

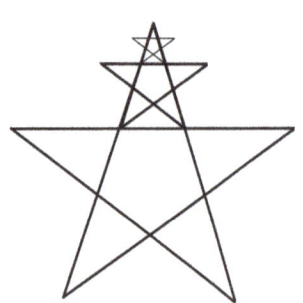 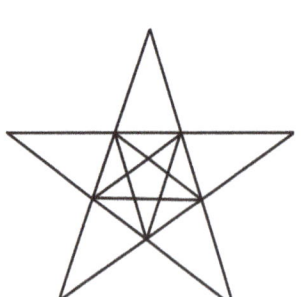 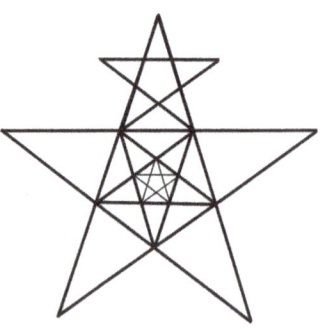

Whilst the entire human body can be perceived as a 5 pointed star, other smaller 5 pointed stars can also be explored relative to the human body. Different orientations of the star elucidate hidden significance and new correspondences.

In the figure opposite the 5 pointed star is orientated to the body so that the lower points of the star are settled into the pelvis with its wealth of unconscious emotion, intuition and creativity. The upper points of the star are seated into the shoulder joints at the chest level where our more conscious hopes, desires and aspirations are to be found, whilst the final point touches up into the throat and the field of expression. The movement of consciousness in the 5 pointed star is inward and upward so this particular orientation symbolises the blending and expression of both conscious and unconscious impulses.

One of the most important lines of symmetry in the human body is at the respiratory diaphragm. The physical correspondences suggested by this orientation of the 5 pointed star are unique. As the movement of consciousness represented by the star is inward and upward, all the organs beneath the line of symmetry at the diaphragm have their correspondences above this line, not by reflection but by translation, they are literally slid or projected upward.

The diagonal aspect of the 5 pointed star pattern creates correspondences in a diagonal orientation, where abdominal organs below the navel on the left side are translated into the upper right side above the diaphragm and vice versa. The digestive organs (liver, gall bladder, stomach, pancreas) above the navel correspond to the upper chest and shoulder areas on the *same* side.

In the vertical aspect, the 5 pointed star pattern creates correspondences of all the organs beneath the diaphragm on the same side above.

Headaches, shoulder pain and sore necks can, of course, be treated by working on the reflex areas in the feet and hands, but a more lasting outcome can be achieved by addressing the cause of these pains, which in many cases start in the organs of digestion, which can be treated by working the 5 pointed star correspondences.

The lower pelvic organs correspond to the breast area. Disturbances in the ovaries can be detected as painful areas over the breasts. The left ovary relates to the right breast area and vice versa. Careful study of the charts overleaf will show many significant correspondences.

> "The existence of pentagons and hexagons doth neatly declare how nature Geometrizeth and observeth order in all things".
> Sir Thomas Browne

Diagonal 5 Pointed Star Correspondences

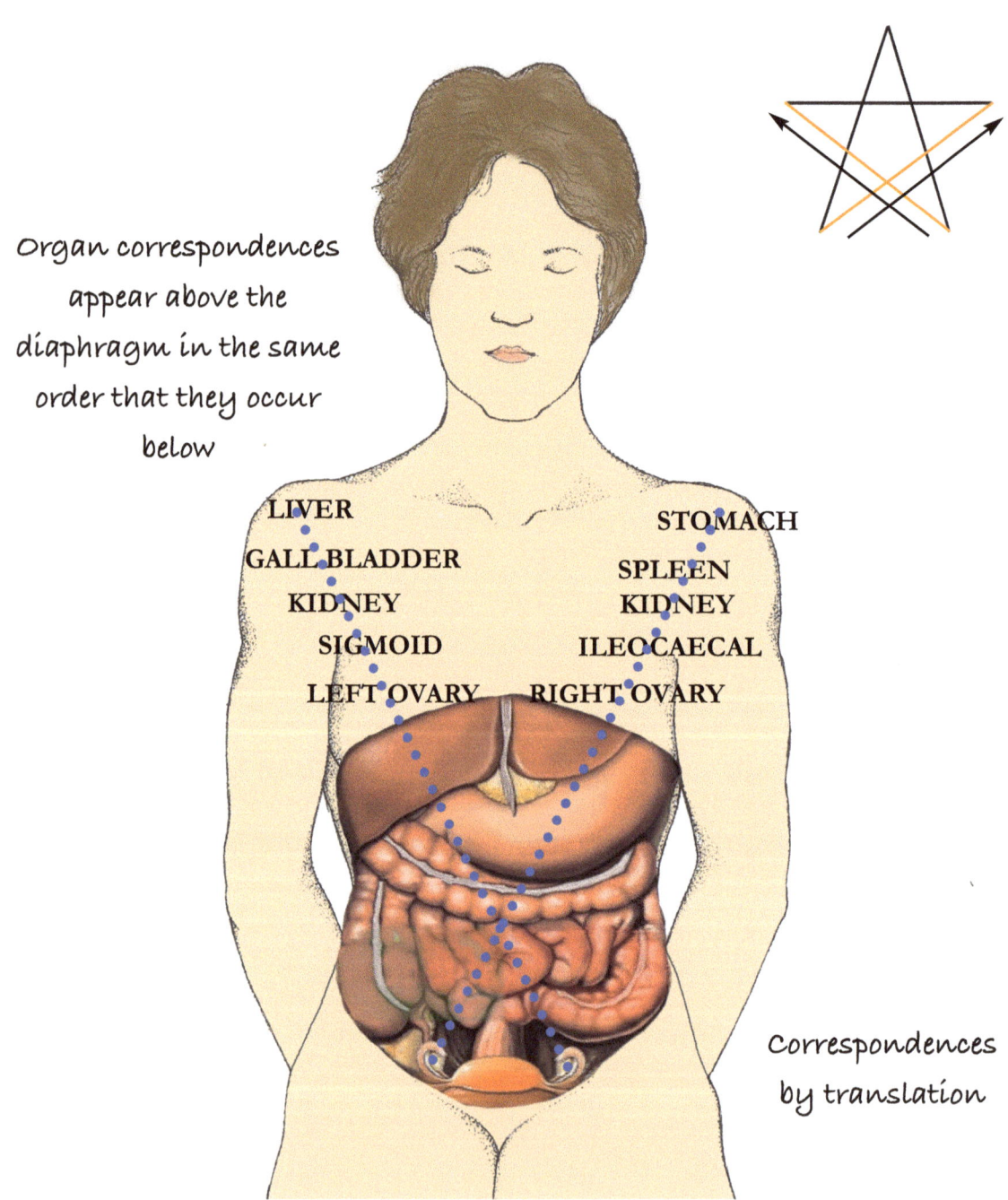

Organ correspondences appear above the diaphragm in the same order that they occur below

LIVER
GALL BLADDER
KIDNEY
SIGMOID
LEFT OVARY

STOMACH
SPLEEN
KIDNEY
ILEOCAECAL
RIGHT OVARY

Correspondences by translation

Vertical 5 Pointed Star Correspondences

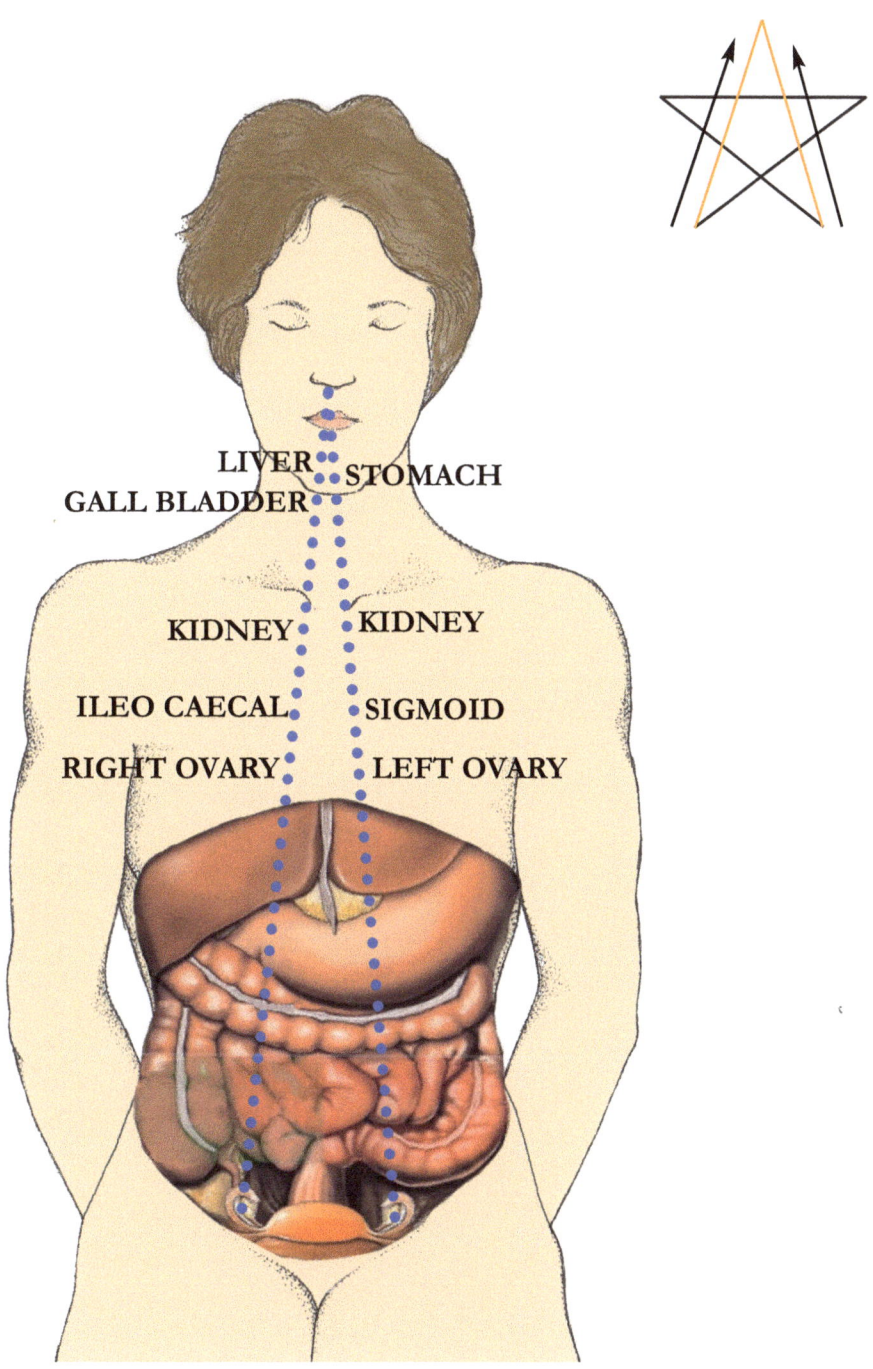

Activating The 5 Pointed Star

It is helpful to activate the whole 5 pointed star before working on any specific correspondences.

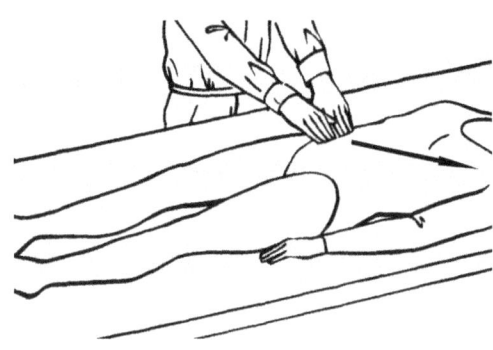

Begin by levelling the finger tips and then pressing gently down into the abdomen over the inguinal ligament. Go as deep as the body will allow, do not use force. Then keeping the fingers at this depth repeatedly scoop up toward the opposite shoulder until the abdomen begins to soften and relax.

N.B. It is important to position your body so that you get a clear diagonal line of application to the opposite shoulder. In the following two techniques the lower hand pushes in a specific direction as shown by the arrows.

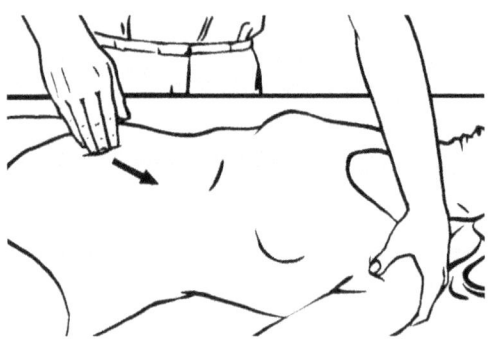

If you begin on the right side of the body leave your right hand on the abdominal contact and move the left hand to the left shoulder joint. Stimulate the shoulder area with circular movements of the thumb paying particular attention to tight areas. Alternate the stimulation until both contacts feel softer and you can feel a good energetic coherence between them.

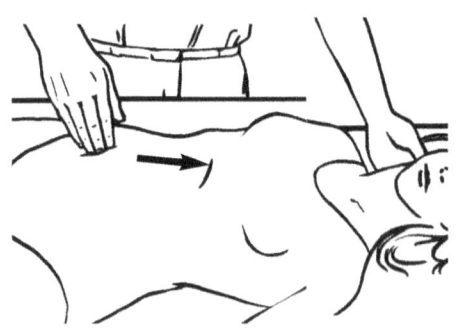

Maintain the lower contact and move the left hand to the back of the neck and work into tension areas in the neck until they too soften and relax. Hold the two contacts and establish a coherent flow between them.

Repeat this entire process on the other side of the body.

Treating 5 Pointed Star Correspondences

LIVER

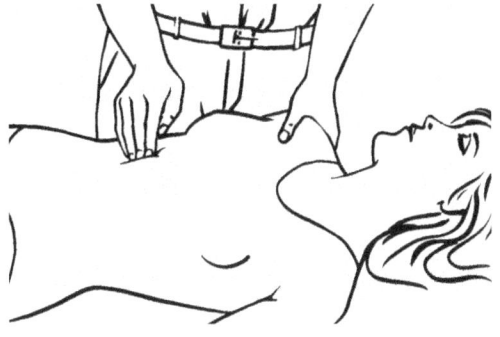

Initially, place the finger pads of the right hand over the liver area. The liver is a very large organ and you will need to work over the whole organ.

Your left hand gently grips the right shoulder joint with the thumb on the front.

Stimulate the shoulder area with circular movements of the thumb, paying particular attention to any areas of tension. Alternate with gentle stimulation over the whole of the liver, then place your hands, palm down, over the two areas until you feel a good degree of energetic coherence between both contacts.

STOMACH

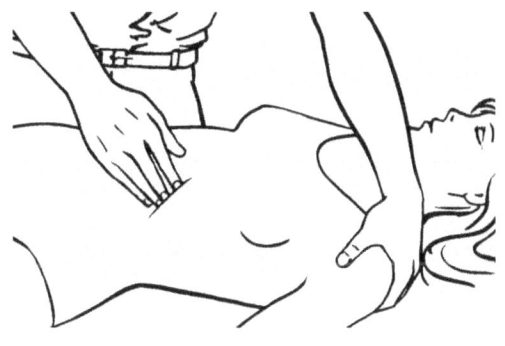

Stomach reflexes can also be worked from the right side of the body but it may be more comfortable to move to the left side. The technique is essentially the same as when working the liver.

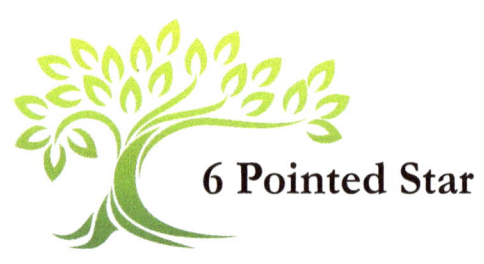
6 Pointed Star

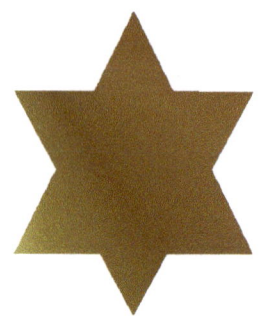

The fundamental symbolism of the 6 pointed star is birth. That is to say, the point at which spirit incarnates into the physical world, but it is also a more general symbol of any kind of birth process.

Physically, the downward pointing triangle, representing the male principle of expansive energy, is expressed in the broad shoulders and narrow pelvis of the male. The upward pointing triangle, representing the female principle of reflection, is expressed as the wider pelvis and relatively narrower shoulder of the female. To some degree, you can see the manifestation of the balance of 6 pointed star, as it was at conception, in the relative size of the hips and pelvis of the mature male and female.

Ultimately, the 6 pointed star is the symbol of any duality within the human being. It can, for example, be seen in the alternating activation of the different branches of autonomic nervous system in the physical body.

In some teachings the male and female aspects of the star, that is to say, which triangle represents male and which female, differ and once again we refer back to the concept of perspective. Taken from the perspective of looking down into matter from spirit, the view looks the reverse of a perspective from matter looking back up to spirit. Hence, from the perspective of the realm of matter, the upward pointing triangle is male and the downward is female, whereas from the realm spirit, the downward pointing triangle is male and the upward is female. Both perspectives are valid.

The 6 pointed star represents unification, the balancing of opposites.

Male - Female

Spirit - Matter

Conscious - Unconscious

Rational - Intuitive

Involution - Evolution

The 6 Pointed Star in Nature

As the 6 pointed star is composed of two triangles it represents balanced structure, strength and stability. As with the 5 pointed star, the 6 pointed star is clearly visible in nature. It is the shape of minimum energy and greatest strength. It can be found in the cells of the human body, the configuration of insects, quartz crystals, wood cellulose, rock, the honeycomb and snowflakes.

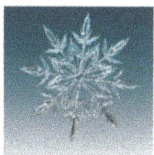

The 6 pointed star is a two dimensional figure composed of two triangles. It can also be perceived in three dimensions as two pyramids.

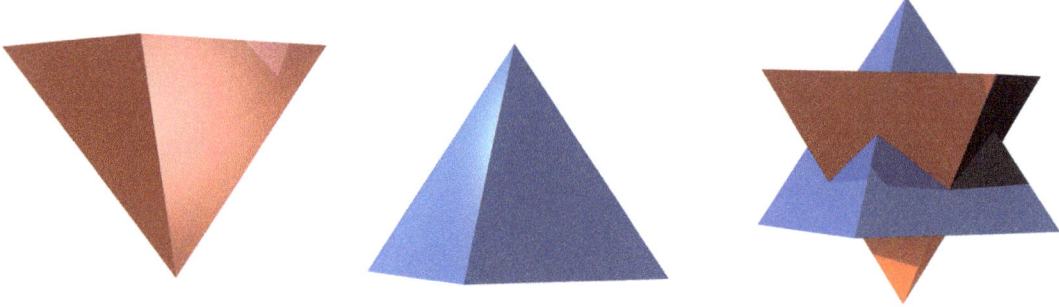

The most widely understood concept symbolised by the 6 pointed star is the juxtaposition of spirit and matter. The downward pointing triangle is representative of spirit involving and manifesting as matter or form whereas the upward pointing triangle is representative of matter or form evolving back to spirit. As such this is a classic example of duality and the forces present in the human being as both matter and spirit. The 6 pointed star can be perceived as indicating the possibility of a perfect balance of opposing forces within us all.

This is a very broad understanding, but if we bring it down to the human level, it is best understood, not as the balance of male and female but as the relationship between individuality and personality. What is meant by individuality is the higher, spiritual or soul self and the personality as the egoic self.

A person on the involutionary phase of existence and experience, dominated by the ego, is represented by the lower upward pointing triangle or pyramid. It is a bottom-heavy structure, deeply settled in the world. A person on the evolutionary path is seeking the sacred in life, something other than the physical and mundane. They do this at a personal level through bringing into their awareness the concept that they have a soul, an essence, a higher self, a type of unique individuality that has its origin in the spiritual realm. This is represented by the downward pointing triangle or pyramid. It is a top-heavy structure that has its roots or foundation in the spiritual world or plane of existence.

However, it is not a matter of shifting to the spiritual and trying to live entirely from that level, as this can ultimately lead to a person who is so spiritual that they are no good here on Earth.

The real evolutionary path seeks to bring heaven and earth, spirit and matter, individuality and personality into a balanced relationship and heralds the development of an evolved human who can move beyond the limitations of the five senses given to us to make sense of our world.

This process creates internal tension, as both living in the mundane physical world, with all its charm and powerful egoic attachments and simultaneously holding to the idea of the existence of a more spiritual or soulful life, with a very different set of values, is a profound challenge.

This process of the reconciliation of opposing forces literally creates internal pressures in the consciousness of a person as they seek to find and express the sacred in the mundane in a meaningful way.

This struggle creates what has been called the 'diamond soul' or 'jewel in the lotus'. A balanced, clear, God and self realised individual, the perfected human being.

In most esoteric traditions, this jewel of transformed consciousness is located in the region of the heart.

Before this process begins, the ordinary human being can be represented by two triangles whose points just touch (Fig. 1). In the beginning phase of this complete process of the spiritualisation of matter and its corollary, the materialisation of spirit, the triangles start to interpenetrate (Fig. 2). As the process deepens and matures, the two triangles or pyramids continue to merge into each other until they finally fully interpenetrate (Fig. 3 and Fig. 4). The perfected human with the jewel inside is represented by the full 6 pointed star (Fig. 5).

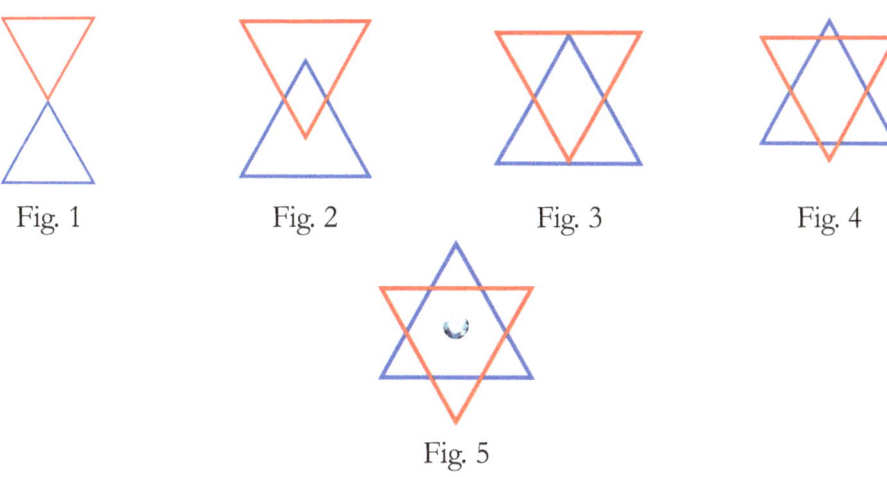

Fig. 1   Fig. 2   Fig. 3   Fig. 4

Fig. 5

During this process, particularly in its early phases, a person will often shift back and forth from one way of being to the other, discovering that when in the consciousness of the lower pyramid, the understanding and perception possible from the upper pyramid is not available to them and vice versa. As the process continues, it becomes possible to blend the two more and more, but it is a challenge as consciousness has a tendency to flip from one to the other. To hold both simultaneously and to crystallise that blended consciousness is a life long journey.

In esoteric terms, this is the initiatory process of moving from being a natural or unillumined man or woman to becoming an illuminated or enlightened being.

To evolve and bring matter and spirit into relationship is, in some sense, against Nature. Nature simply is, with its cycles of birth and decay. Human beings serve Nature through simply living, reproducing and dying.

This whole process can be thought of as two rivers or streams in life, one stream involutionary the other evolutionary.

An individual in the evolutionary stream, who can be perceived as a droplet of water within it, is subject to all manner of influences upon its movement. Yet, from the perspective of its personality or ego it feels important in itself. It feels as if its life matters. It imagines it is doing something yet, in reality, it is simply following the dictates of the stream. In this first stream, the individual is actually unimportant, overall there is a destiny in terms of the stream as a whole but not in terms of the experience of the individual droplets that make up the stream. They simply flow with the current.

However, there is another stream flowing nearby, the evolutionary one. Occasionally, as a droplet comes to the surface in the involutionary stream, it sees the other evolutionary stream and wonders about it. As its curiosity grows, it is granted more glimpses of the evolutionary stream and begins to wonder if it can get across to it. In turbulent water, a droplet is sometimes thrown up and out of the involutionary stream only to fall back into it. Yet, from this experience arises the idea that there may be the possibility to move across to the other stream. The concept of the freedom to choose is born within the individual that is that droplet.

Yet, before a crossing is possible an individual must die to the first river, a death in life that ultimately can lead to a rebirth.

As Jesus said:

"I say unto thee, Except a man be born again, he cannot see the kingdom of God".

"Except a man be born of water and of the Spirit, he cannot enter into the kingdom of God. That which is born of the flesh is flesh; and that which is born of the Spirit is spirit.

Marvel not that I said unto thee, Ye must be born again. The wind bloweth where it listeth, and thou hearest the sound thereof, but canst not tell whence it cometh, and whither it goeth: so is every one that is born of the Spirit".

John 3 - King James Bible

This death is not physical, but the enormous reduction in the pull of the current in the first river upon the individual droplet; a reduction in the charm of all that this river has to offer. Thus, allowing the individual droplet to pass over to the other stream at the right moment.

In this other evolutionary stream, the individual droplet truly does matter and can have a personal destiny governed by the nature of its essence as opposed to its personality.

This metaphor only takes us so far, as true illumination requires the building of a bridge, called by some the rainbow bridge. This allows the movement of the individual droplet from one stream to the other at will and ultimately the possibility of staying on the apex of the bridge. From this vantage point, both streams can be perceived at the same time and any movement from one stream to the other can be timed perfectly, in accord to the conditions present in each.

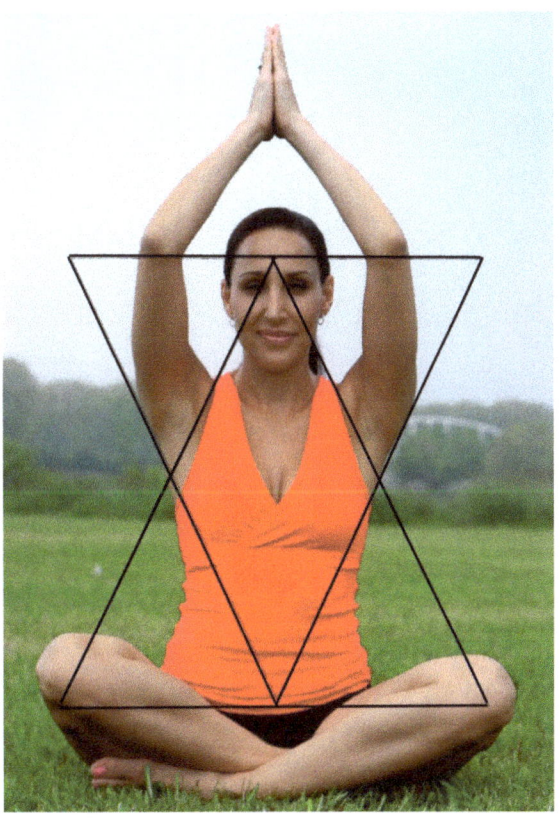

Practical Work on the 6 Pointed Star

The 6 pointed star extends beyond the body. When working with the 6 pointed star it is important to understand that it exists as a vibrating pattern in the energetic body and the auric field. The auric field is the name given to the radiance that emits from the human energy body. By way of analogy, if you think of an old style electrical heater in which a bare wire is wrapped around a ceramic core, when a current of electricity is passed through the wire it begins to glow. The glow is both radiant light and heat. The human energy body acts in a similar way in that as the life energy flows through it, it gives off a radiance.

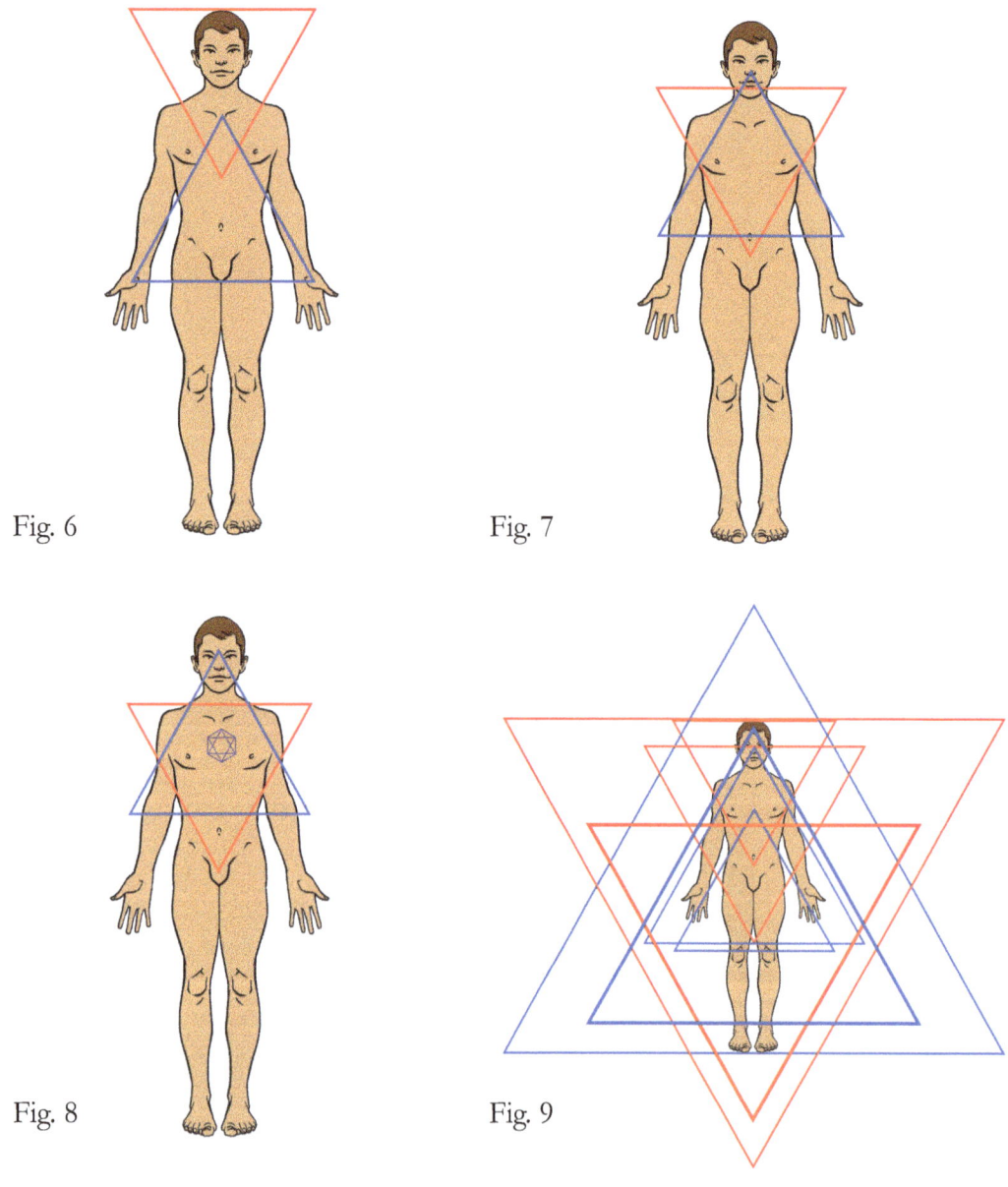

Fig. 6

Fig. 7

Fig. 8

Fig. 9

Figures 6 and 7 show some of the different degrees of interaction of the two interlaced triangles or pyramids when superimposed on the human body. Figure 8 showns the fully interlaced structures with the diamond soul or the jewel in the lotus in the chest. Figure 9 shows multiple interlaced 6 pointed star structures of varying sizes. Stars within stars. The size of the stars could be seen to represent different levels of the expansion of consciousness.

A specific orientation of the 6 pointed star is to view the downward pointing triangle. or pyramid, as relating to the head, with the base at the third eye and the upward pointing triangle, or pyramid, relating to the pelvis, with its base at the symphysis pubis. In Polarity Therapy, Dr Randolph Stone focused on this orientation of the 6 pointed star to the body. He saw its resonances mostly in terms of structural relationship and the reflected correspondences between the head and pelvis (see fig. 10 and 11).

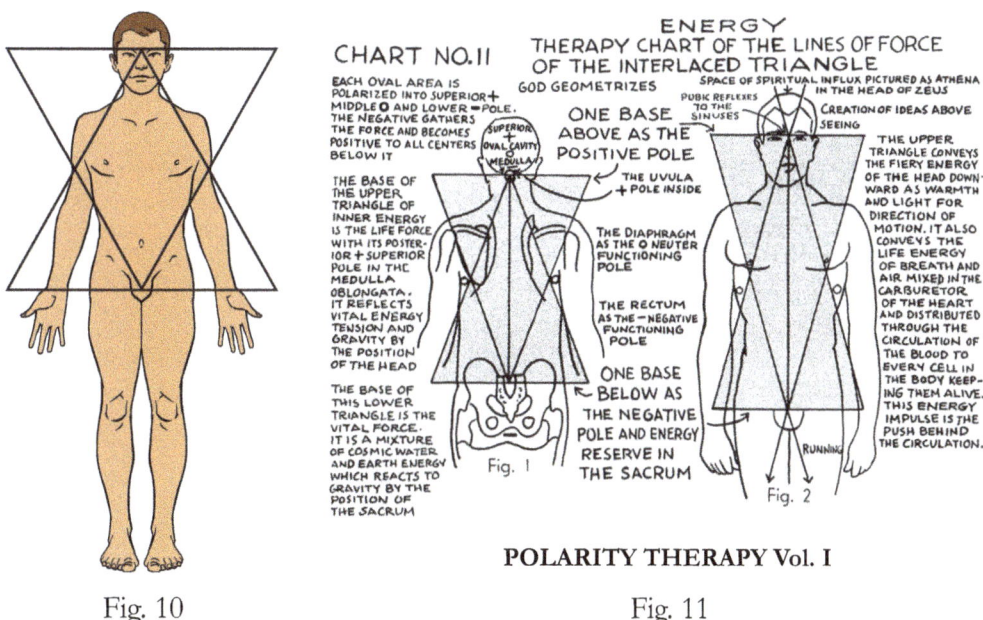

Fig. 10   Fig. 11

In Holonomic Reflexology, the focus on this pattern also uses this same level of interpenetration, but not in terms of structure but to stabilise what it represents in terms of the initiatory journey. For most on this journey, having achieved a connection between the involutionary and evolutionary aspects of the human initiatory experience, there is always a tendency to flip from one to the other. This is the most common experience for anyone on a spiritual path, experiencing all the challenges of acknowledging and expressing the reality of existing as a spiritual being in a physical, earthly incarnation.

The practical work on the 6 pointed star is used to stabilise the interconnectedness of the two pyramids or triangles and, at the end of the session, the practitioner's focus is on the germinal jewel in the lotus at the heart level.

Activating The 6 Pointed Star

Activating the 6 pointed star will help to bring about balance in a client who is struggling with any of the major dualities in life. It is important to tune into the pattern which extends beyond the physical body. Ideally, the two pyramids should extend equidistantly. If one pyramid, or even just one side of a pyramid, extends only a little from the body then it will be necessary to encourage it out further. Working the 6 pointed star requires an acute sensitivity to the life energy as much of the time one hand is in the auric field tracing the boundaries of the pyramids.

The Lower Pyramid

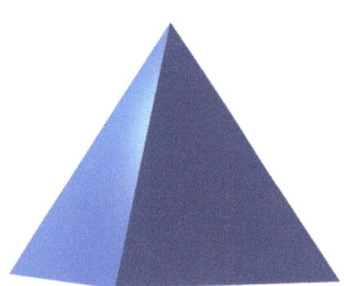

Standing at the client's right side, place the left thumb on the third eye above the bridge of the nose and the right hand on the hip joint.

Tune into the energy at the hip joint and then slowly draw you hand away from the body maintaining a connection to the energy. At some point there will feel a slight resistance to the movement, or other subtle changes which usually indicate that the pattern has reached full expansion. Then move to the other side of the client and placing the right thumb on the third eye and the left hand at the hip draw out the energy from the hip ensuring that it matches the other side.

To address the three dimensionality of the pyramid, leave the right thumb on the third eye and have the left hand directly above the pubic bone, sensing the frontal plane of the pyramid.

The Upper Pyramid

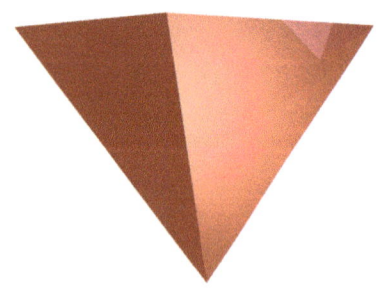

The technique for the upper triangle is the same. This time the contacts consist of a thumb contact at the centre of the pubic bone and a hand contact to the side of the head over the ear and TMJ. Once again establish a connection at each contact and then slowly draw out the upper pyramid on both sides. Then make a connection above the head sensing the frontal plane if the upper pyramid. It is important to establish a synchronicity between the upper and lower Pyramids.

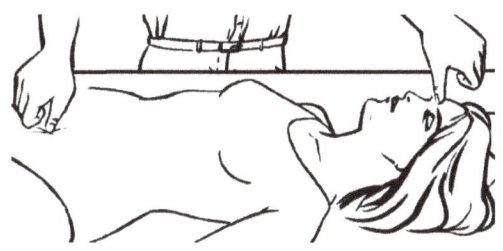

Standing at the client's right side, connect the third eye to the centre of the pubic bone using the thumbs. Use a focused intent to visualise two similarly sized pyramids interpenetrating and forming a perfect three dimensional 6 pointed star pattern.

Finally, shift the focus to the heart and visualise the nascent jewel in the lotus that is beginning to form there.

> "Man's threefold lower nature—consisting of his physical organism, his emotional nature, and his mental faculties—reflects the light of his threefold Divinity and bears witness of It in the physical world. Man's three bodies are symbolized by an upright triangle; his threefold spiritual nature by an inverted triangle. These triangles symbolize the spiritual and material universes linked together in the constitution of the human creature, who partakes of both Nature and Divinity. Man's animal nature partakes of the earth; his divine nature of the heavens; his human nature of the mediator".
> *The Secret Teachings of All Ages* - Manly P. Hall - 1928

Final Thoughts

It could be said that this book on Holonomic Reflexology explores the concept of 'The Big Picture'. It provides an expansive view on the nature of the interconnected aspects of the human being and the connection with the greater forces at play beyond every day consciousness.

It speaks to the wonder of the Creation that we are all an integral part of, unites us with the many networks of consciousness at play in our Universe and, in some small way, re-ignites a spark within us; an eternal flame that reminds us that we are a unique facet in the jewel that is our Universe.

To get the most from this book it is necessary to embrace the concepts behind the reflexes and not merely regard the maps and reflex charts as a way of treating by rote or simply as a way of joining all the dots. The effort involved in a deeper study will reward therapist and client beyond measure.

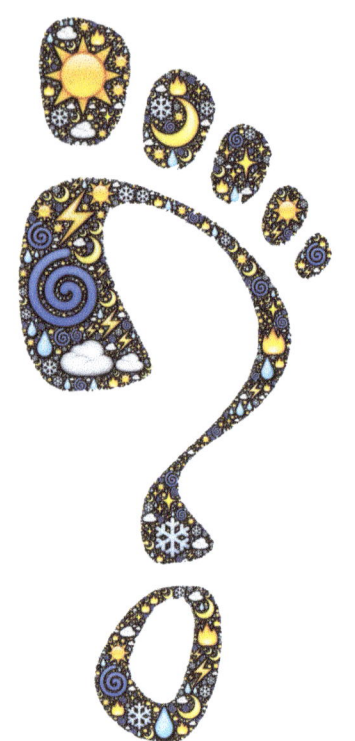

Morag Campbell and **Phil Young** are directors of Masterworks International, a training consultancy for Polarity Therapy. They have run trainings and workshops around the world since the 1980s and were instrumental in the establishment of the International Polarity Education Alliance. They have written the following books related to their chosen field.

POLARITY THERAPY—HEALING WITH LIFE ENERGY Alan Siegel and Phil Young

POLARITY THERAPY– where ENERGY meets STRUCTURE and FUNCTION Phil Young

QUINTA ESSENTIA - THE FIVE ELEMENTS Morag Campbell

DON'T START WHAT YOU CAN'T FINISH –THE BOOK OF COMPLETION Morag Campbell

Bibliography

Polarity Therapy Vol I and II by Dr. Randolph Stone - Book Publishing Co

Health Building by Dr. Randolph. Stone - Book Publishing Co

Symmetry by Hermann Weyl - Princeton University Press 1952

Symmetry: A Very Short Introduction by Ian Stewart - Oxford University Press 2013

The Symmetries of Things by John H. Conway, Heidi Burgiel, and Chaim Goodman-Strauss - A K Peters/CRC Press 2008

Richard Feynman - http://www.feynmanlectures.caltech.edu/I_52.html

Image Credits

Cover And Theory

Seated Forward bend - Elena Ray

Tree Icon Concept - Christos Georghiou

Young brunette - photoeuphoria

Zodiac Signs - maria am

Energy flows - Michael Nolan

Zen Stones - Dimitrovavalentina

Yin Yang Human - Rolffimages

Finger pointing at hand - Linda Garland

Body Bliss - Elena Ray

Sleeping Woman's feet - Andystjohm

Cartography

Body Outline figures - Michael Nolan

Anatomy, Muscles and Skeleton - Dusan Todorovic

Male Human Skeleton - Leorello Calvetti

Human Lungs and Trachea - Igor Tokalenko

Urinary Bladder and Kidneys - Guniita

Human Skull - Oguzaral

Esoteric Correspondences

Starfish on rocks - solarseven

Geranium flower - yury Shirokov

Sliced Apple with pips star centre - Vrabpeter 1

Close Up of Dog Rose - Richard Griffin

Diamond Soul - Morag Campbell

Interlaced star - Morag Campbell

Witch Hazel - photographieundmehr

Peas in a pod - Robert Hyrons

Fresh half orange - Marazem

Smoky quartz crystal - Sorsillo

Polarity massage - Erik de Graaf

For further reading on Polarity Therapy we recommend the following titles

POLARITY THERAPY

Healing with Life Energy

Alan Siegel ND and Phil Young PTP

An excellent practical introduction to Polarity including the principles that underlie the work and clear treatment protocols

ISBN: 978-0-9544450-5-8

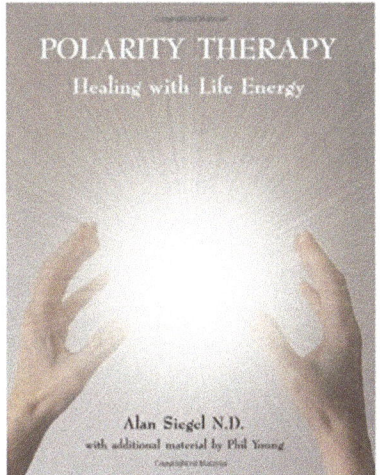

POLARITY THERAPY

Where Energy meets Structure and Function

Phil Young PTP

A more advanced look at Polarity with special emphasis on the dynamics of structure and the effects of gravity on the body

ISBN: 978-0-9933465-2-1

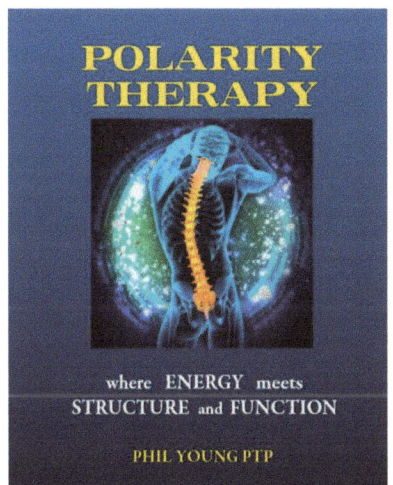

For Workshops and Training in Polarity Therapy and Holonomic Reflexology

Web site: www.masterworksinternational.com

Email: info@masterworksinternational.com

For further reading on Polarity Therapy we recommend the following titles

POLARITY THERAPY

Healing with Life Energy

Alan Siegel ND and Phil Young PTP

An excellent practical introduction to Polarity including the principles that underlie the work and clear treatment protocols

ISBN: 978-0-9544450-5-8

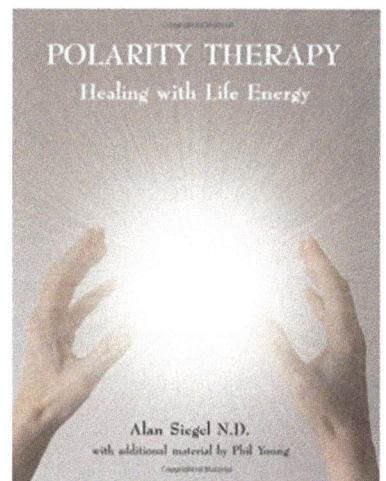

POLARITY THERAPY

Where Energy meets Structure and Function

Phil Young PTP

A more advanced look at Polarity with special emphasis on the dynamics of structure and the effects of gravity on the body

ISBN: 978-0-9933465-2-1

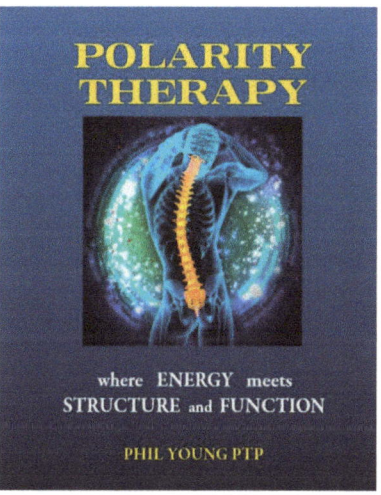

For Workshops and Training in Polarity Therapy and Holonomic Reflexology

Web site: www.masterworksinternational.com

Email: info@masterworksinternational.com

www.ingramcontent.com/pod-product-compliance
Lightning Source LLC
Chambersburg PA
CBHW051548220426
43671CB00021B/2978